Praise for
Yes, Thank You

In *Yes, Thank You: Tapping Into the Superpower of Gratitude*, EFT Master Carol Look offers a deeply personal and profoundly insightful exploration of how gratitude can transform our lives. By weaving together personal stories, EFT Tapping, and inspiring testimonials, this book provides a comprehensive guide to overcoming obstacles and embracing a more positive, resilient mindset. The 30-Day gratitude challenge offers readers a structured path to integrating gratitude into their daily routines. This book is an invaluable resource for anyone looking to unlock the full potential of gratitude and live a more joyful, fulfilling life.

Dr. Peta Stapleton, Clinical & Health Psychologist
Professor, Bond University, Australia
www.evidencebasedeft.com

What if gratitude is the key to truly thriving—but hidden emotional blocks are standing in your way? In *Yes, Thank You*, Carol Look compassionately guides you to clear these barriers, transforming daily gratitude from a 'nice idea' into a life-changing practice. By following her proven process, you'll create lasting space for deeper joy, greater peace, and authentic emotional freedom.

Rick Wilkes, Emotional Freedom Coach
www.thrivingnow.com

I've had the privilege of witnessing Carol teach hundreds of people from all over the world about the science and power of gratitude. I'm so grateful she finally wrote this deeply inspiring book, *Yes, Thank You*, that will continue to be a source of inner healing and inspiration to many. When you learn how to experience and cultivate gratitude, it will transform your heart and life in every way. Carol is a living testament to this.

Roos van der Blom, Functional Medicine Practitioner
Founder of DNA Care www.dnacare.nl

Yes, Thank You is a beautiful blend of honesty, wisdom, and possibility. Carol Look acknowledges life's challenges while showing us that gratitude can be a true superpower. With clarity and compassion, she offers insights and healing tools to help us release the past and step into a more joyful future. Carol's work is transformational, and this book is going to inspire and uplift so many lives!

Julie Fedeli, Best-Selling Co-author, *Midlife Upgrade*
www.midlifeupgrade.com

The impact of Carol Look's teachings on my life has been immeasurable, and I'm thrilled she has finally written *Yes, Thank You* so others can benefit from her gratitude work. With her classic laser-sharp clarity, she has combined the often painful truth about life's hardships with the potential and promise of tapping into the superpower of gratitude. Her insights will bring hope and healing opportunities for readers who want to let go of the past and create a joyful future.

Leslie Vellios, LCSW, Advanced EFT Coach
www.stresslesswitheft.com

Carol Look's work has been transformative in my healing journey, and her illuminating new book *Yes, Thank You* is no exception. Carol weaves her childhood challenges with healing exercises and science-backed reasons to tap into the superpower of gratitude. This book and Carol's 30-Day Gratitude Challenge are a must for anyone who is serious about wanting to invite more happiness and joy in their lives.

    Carissa Brockman, MACP, CCC – Intuitive Somatic Coach
    www.carissabrockman.com

Carol Look's expert guidance and clarity on how to tap into the transformative power of gratitude is nothing short of life-changing. I was skeptical at first, but her simple, effective use of the Tapping Technique made it easy – and the results were undeniable. Carol combines her decades of professional wisdom with authentic compassion, leading us gently and powerfully into healing and abundance. *Yes, Thank You* is a must-have for anyone ready to shift their energy and embrace a life of gratitude.

    Audrey Faust, Best-Selling Author, *She Grows Rich*
    www.audreyfaustconsulting.com

In this compelling book, *Yes, Thank You,* Carol Look blends scientific research and personal stories with practical EFT Sequences, offering a powerful blueprint to supercharge a daily gratitude practice. *Yes, Thank You* is a must-read for anyone looking to elevate their life through the power of gratitude!

    Alissa Smith, Intuitive Counselor, Spiritual Mentor
    www.alissasmithintuitive.com

I'm thrilled that Carol finally put her gratitude work in her new book, *Yes, Thank You* so a wider audience will be able to improve all aspects of their lives. I can't even begin to count the number of blocks Carol has helped me release. She taught me the power of deep gratitude—not just a surface-level 'I'm thankful.' I continue to use her Gratitude Tapping to this day.

Gretchen Pritts, www.calminglittleminds.com

YES,
THANK YOU

YES, THANK YOU

Tapping Into the Superpower of Gratitude

CAROL LOOK
LCSW, Founding EFT Master

Yes, Thank You
Copyright © 2025 Carol Look

All rights reserved. No part of this publication may be reproduced, distributed, or transmitted in any form or by any electronic or mechanical means, including photocopying, recording, or information storage and retrieval systems, without prior written permission in writing of Thought Leader Academy Publishing, or its duly authorized agent, except in the case of brief quotations embodied in reviews and certain other non-commercial uses permitted by copyright law.
For information regarding permission, contact the publisher.

Paperback ISBN: 979-8-9922573-8-0

Disclaimer: The information contained in this book is for educational and informational purposes only and is not intended as medical or psychological advice. Emotional Freedom Techniques (EFT) or "Tapping" is a self-help tool intended to promote emotional well-being. It is not a substitute for professional medical, psychological, or psychiatric care. Always seek the advice of a qualified healthcare provider with any questions you may have regarding a medical or mental health condition. The author and publisher disclaim any liability for any loss or injury incurred directly or indirectly from the use or application of the techniques described in this book.

Dedication

To my parents, Charlotte and David.
I have always felt grateful for the incredible bond we shared.
Thank you for your love, humor, and depth.
The way you believed in me made everything possible.

Table of Contents

Author's Note 1
Introduction 3

PART ONE
MY STORY

CHAPTER 1
My Blocks 19

PART TWO
THE PROBLEM

CHAPTER 2
The Costs 43

CHAPTER 3
The Payoff 54

PART THREE
THE SOLUTION

CHAPTER 4
All About EFT Tapping 73

CHAPTER 5
Your Container Is Full 89

CHAPTER 6
Low Self-Esteem 108

CHAPTER 7
Self-Sabotaging Behavior 124

CHAPTER 8
Health Challenges 147

PART FOUR
STORIES AND INVITATIONS

CHAPTER 9
Before and After Stories — 165

CHAPTER 10
Gratitude Invitations — 175

PART FIVE
THE CHALLENGE

CHAPTER 11
30-Day Gratitude Challenge — 183

Conclusion — 218

Endnotes — 219

Gratitude — 224

About the Author — 226

Author's Note

Emotional Freedom Techniques (EFT) (often referred to simply as "Tapping" or "EFT Tapping" in this book) is gaining scientific support, but please note that it is still considered experimental in nature. All readers are required to take full responsibility for their physical and mental health, and their use of EFT or Tapping for any psychological, emotional, or physical challenges.

The material in this book is educational in nature and is not intended to be a substitute for traditional medical care, assessment, diagnosis, therapy, or advice and treatment from a health care professional.

Neither EFT nor any of the information in this book is intended to be used to diagnose, treat, cure, or prevent any disease or disorder. If after using the Tapping exercises in this book you feel overwhelmed with emotion or you remember past events or previously forgotten memories that are disturbing, it is your responsibility to seek professional help from your medical doctor, your therapist, mental health counselor, or a trained and experienced EFT practitioner.

All names and identifying details of clients have been changed to protect their privacy. *Unless I received express permission from a client to share the details of their journey, the stories you will read in* Yes, Thank You *are amalgams of clients, friends, family members, and colleagues I have had the honor of working with in my practice.*

*Tell me, what is it
you plan to do with your
one wild and precious life?*

**Mary Oliver,
"The Summer Day"**[1]

Introduction

If you knew that consistently expressing gratitude could lower your stress levels by 28%, would you ***start a gratitude practice?***[2]

If you knew that in an analysis of 30 sleep studies, 60% determined that regularly expressing gratitude improved both sleep quality and duration for participants, would you ***commit to a gratitude practice now?***[3]

If you knew that practicing gratitude could increase your happiness by 25%, would that be the inspiration you need to finally ***stick to a gratitude practice?***[4]

Research shows that when trust increases in a romantic relationship, more than 50% of that increase is linked to gratitude.[5] Maybe that statistic would encourage you to set your alarm 10 minutes earlier every morning and start a gratitude practice immediately.

I'm not suggesting that using a steady practice of gratitude is the fountain of health and happiness...

Or am I?

Dr. Joe Dispenza conducted a study in which he asked participants to practice feeling gratitude 15 minutes a day for four days. After the four days, his participants increased an antibody that plays a vital role in our immune system, Immunoglobulin A, by over 50%.[6]

Regularly expressing gratitude can mimic a pharmaceutical; a study with *more than 25,000 participants* showed a significant association between gratitude and lower hypertension risk.[7] Other times gratitude acts like a psychotherapist, helping you improve your self-esteem and your relationship satisfaction. And still other times it acts like technology and can upgrade your processor. But if it's not a medication, a psychotherapist, or technology, then what is it?

*Gratitude is an emotion,
a mood, an attitude, and as the research shows,
a superpower for your body, mind, and spirit.*

And it's available to everyone.

Like any self-care habit, a gratitude practice is a behavior you engage in regularly, a habit you feel committed to as part of your self-care routine. You wouldn't skip it once you've woven it into your day because the benefits far outweigh the effort.

Gratitude practices are recommended in numerous self-help programs, in popular books, and as a means to *change the channel* when you're heading down a dark or unproductive alley.

*What if expressing gratitude
can rewire your brain?*

Sixty-four randomized clinic trials showed that gratitude improved both depression and anxiety symptoms – a statistic that Big Pharma would not want you to know.[8] The research also found that expressing gratitude lowers your cortisol levels by 23%[9] and lowers your risk of developing chronic health conditions. In fact, gratitude lowers the risk of cardiovascular disease by a whopping 15%.[10] Psychiatrist and Director of the Center on Stress and Health at Stanford Medicine, Dr. David Spiegel, said that the study's message was:

**Count your blessings, and you'll
have more time to count your years.**[11]

Numerous studies, including one cited by Penn Medicine Princeton Health, revealed that while expressing and receiving gratitude, "the brain releases dopamine and serotonin."[12] Dopamine is the reward chemical, and serotonin is the happiness chemical. What are the effects of releasing these chemicals into your brain and body? The primary stress hormone, cortisol, decreases, immune function increases, and happiness levels improve.

Chasing happiness is a BIG business in our world today. What if the means to achieving happiness has been right under our noses the whole time?

In numerous articles about the *neuroscience of gratitude*, evidence shows that thanks to neuroplasticity, expressing gratitude literally rewires our brain.

A study showed that almost 80% of employees are more motivated to be productive when they feel appreciated.[13] I feel quite certain that most of my former bosses never knew this.

Knowing these scientific facts might change your calculation around whether you're going to simply dabble in expressing gratitude, or commit to starting a daily practice.

> *Did I mention that engaging in a gratitude practice is FREE?*

No special equipment, no intensive time commitment, and no expensive training or certifications. Just pick up a pen and piece of paper and you can get started.

It should come as no surprise that extremely successful people keep a gratitude practice too. Self-help guru Tony Robbins has been interviewed talking about "priming his day" with expressing gratitude. Oprah Winfrey reports writing in her daily gratitude journal. Brené Brown is quoted saying:

> *I don't have to chase extraordinary moments to find happiness – it's right in front of me if I'm paying attention and practicing gratitude.*
>
> **Brené Brown**[14]

I didn't write this book because I was perfect at sticking to a gratitude practice. I wrote it because I wasn't. First, I had to learn which gratitude practices worked for me, and then I had to feel inspired enough to be consistent. I needed a reason to stick to it, to counter all the excuses I used to forget my practice, starting with *life got in the way.*

If I had known that maintaining a consistent gratitude practice would have given me all the science-backed benefits as well as reduced the risk of early mortality, I might have started earlier with my regular practice and been better about keeping it up.

Or would I?

When the scientific research is so prolific, you might find it puzzling as to why you wouldn't follow through with tapping into such an incredible superpower. Why would we turn away from taking care of ourselves with such a simple habit when the results are backed by science?

> ***Because we all have emotional blocks,***
> ***limiting beliefs, and self-sabotaging behaviors***
> ***that eclipse the priority of taking care of ourselves***
> ***and limit our capacity for joy and contentment.***

After more than 30 years of working in the mental health field, I have found three primary blocks that limit our capacity for more joy, contentment, and happiness.

1. <u>There's no more room for joy and contentment</u>. Our emotional container is already too full of negative conflicts and memories from our past.

2. <u>We don't feel deserving of more happiness and fulfillment</u>. As a result of these past emotional conflicts and experiences, we developed low self-esteem, which led us to devalue ourselves.

3. <u>We sabotage our efforts to be happier and more successful</u>. In an attempt to protect ourselves from standing out or being a target for criticism and jealousy, we sabotage our personal and professional success. These behaviors keep us under the radar, and therefore, safe, and out of the spotlight.

If we are emotionally full of the past, don't feel deserving of success and happiness, and are afraid of what feeling better and living an exceptional life might trigger in others, we won't feel inspired to stick to healthy habits and behaviors, much less engage in the superpower of a gratitude practice – ***no matter how astonishing the research is.***

> *The real question is:*
> *How much joy and happiness can you handle?*

Keeping a gratitude practice offers a surefire opportunity to increase your happiness, lower your stress levels, boost your self-esteem, and improve your health. And yet...millions of people, maybe you, are not taking advantage of this superpower on a daily basis. Those three primary blocks keep us locked into a setpoint or comfort zone. We stick within the bounds of what is familiar and safe, and we do everything in our power to avoid rocking the boat.

My passion is helping people like you empty your container of old emotional conflicts, boost your self-esteem, and release the reasons you engage in self-sabotaging behavior. As a psychotherapist with extensive experience in the mental health field, I have witnessed clients repeatedly put the brakes on their progress just as they start to feel better. They neglect the very practices they've been engaged in that have allowed them to feel more joy and fulfillment. They relapse, call the old abusive boyfriend, start overeating, forget to express their gratitude, or avoid the gym. Why? *Because feeling better is:*

> *Impossible when your container is too full,*
> *unattainable when you have low self-esteem,*
> *and unsafe when you don't want to be a target.*

Emotional Math

Success is not an accident. The results that show up in your life come from your emotional responses to life's events, the inherited and hidden beliefs you adopted, and the behaviors you keep choosing.

I can state and restate the benefits of expressing gratitude all day long, but the truth is:

> *You are limiting how much joy and happiness*
> *you can tolerate because you don't have room*
> *for more, don't think you deserve to enjoy more,*
> *and don't feel safe embracing more.*

When we clear our blocks to handling more happiness and contentment, only then are we open to engaging with the superpower of gratitude more fully.

The late great Bob Proctor was often quoted saying:

> *Your why has to be*
> *greater than your why not.*

No matter how emotionally enthusiastic you are about starting a gratitude practice, no matter how big your **why** is after reading the research statistics, **if you haven't dealt with the major blocks to happiness and fulfilment, your why nots will win.**

Your **why** can be a deep desire to attract all sorts of positive results into your life, but if your emotional conflicts (your container is too full), your limiting beliefs (you don't deserve more), and your behavior (self-sabotage) don't change, you can't tolerate more happiness and success, and if you do, you won't be able to maintain it.

> *If your feelings, beliefs*
> *and behaviors don't change,*
> *your results won't change.*

Your blocks will keep you from getting the benefits of the practices, habits, or systems you're trying to implement in your life. If you're not sticking to a daily gratitude practice after hearing the impressive research, you have too many *why nots* in the way.

Why would you not have availed yourself of this free superpower? Most people would say it's about discipline, but it's not. Part of you wants to reap the benefits, but another part of you is afraid of the results. You may be asking yourself:

*What part of me wouldn't want to
tap into this superpower of gratitude,
and feel better every day?*

Good question…the answer might be:

- The part of me that is too preoccupied with old family pain. (There's no room for more happiness and joy.)
- The part of me that has low self-esteem and takes care of others instead of myself. (I don't deserve more happiness and fulfillment.)
- The part of me that wants to sabotage my success in order to stay emotionally safe and under the radar. (Being happier and more fulfilled is unsafe.)

If you use the superpower of gratitude, you will notice positive changes in all areas of your life. Sounds wonderful, right? So what's the catch? Here's the tricky part: when your life improves in one or more areas, your emotional, physical, and financial success will inevitably *rock the boat* with people at work, in your social circle, or in your family. Rocking the boat can be emotionally uncomfortable at best. And if you're not willing to tolerate *their* reactions to your success, or you feel too uncomfortable with feeling noticeably better, that's a good enough reason to "forget" to follow your gratitude practice.

- If you empty your container of all the old past conflicts and are visibly happier, what might be the consequence if a family member notices your improvement? Will this rock the boat or disrupt the equilibrium in the relationship?
- What if you start boosting your self-esteem, saying no, and setting clearer boundaries at work and at home? Whose boat will that rock in your life?
- What if you resolve your need for emotional safety and protection, and let go of habits that have kept you playing small? Then what?

Yes, Thank You • 9

Not everyone will be happy for you. Sad, but true. So when you stick to your gratitude practice, you'll improve your immune system, boost your mood, lower your stress response, and be more optimistic, and then people around you are going to notice those changes. Those people are going to have reactions to those changes, and you're going to have reactions to their reactions!

The benefits of tapping into the superpower of gratitude are crystal clear: better health, improved mood and immune system functioning, general happiness, better sleep, increased relationship satisfaction, and lower blood pressure, to name only a few. There are also studies showing the positive impact of gratitude on everything from diabetes, cholesterol levels, and stroke, to cancer, heart disease, and dementia![15]

What stops you from enjoying these benefits is also clear: your capacity for the joy, contentment, and emotional health that gratitude offers is limited by your blocks.

If you feel defeated by your stops and starts with any habits that are good for you, clearing the blocks is the key to smoothing the path. And clearing your blocks is the key to tapping into the superpower of gratitude, effortlessly, on a regular basis.

So now what?

> *You need to pick the best tool to*
> *clear the blocks, so you can*
> *tap into the superpower of gratitude.*

In this book, I'm going to teach you how to use EFT, the best tool I've found to clear the blocks that limit us from using a gratitude practice. Like gratitude, EFT has the ability to rewire your brain and your nervous system, and has the science to back it.

EFT, or Tapping, is an emotional technology tool that will calm down the fight or flight response in your brain that gets triggered when you're focusing on a thought or memory that feels threatening. This will allow you to empty your container of painful memories, start putting yourself first, and embrace the success you deserve.

Why I Wrote This Book

I have been in the mental health field for three decades, which means that in addition to weathering the losses and hardships I've endured in my own family, I've witnessed stories of grief, destruction, and pain in thousands of clients. I've worked with clients who've lost children, clients who fled war-torn countries, clients from three wars who annihilated others because their lives depended on following orders. I've worked with clients who have been abused physically, sexually, and emotionally. I have been honored to *hold the emotional space* for people's confusion, pain, and unspeakable grief.

I wrote this book because I recognize how hard it is to start and stick to practices that support you feeling good on every level. I also wrote this book because in all my years in the mental health field, I haven't found a better tool than EFT, or Tapping, to clear the blocks that are in your way.

There is a lot to appreciate in life and in this world. Everywhere. But we need to look for it, focus on it, and pay attention to it.

What's the Urgency?

The medical and mental health fallout from our rocketing levels of stress is at an all-time high. The CDC reports that suicide rates increased 37% between 2000 and 2022[16] and WebMD reported that between 75-90% of all doctor's office visits are for stress-related complaints.[17] Addictions are rampant despite impressive improvements in addiction treatment. This isn't a coincidence. What it points to is that whether our stress levels are legitimately increasing or not, we're not managing them effectively.

The simplicity and potency of keeping a gratitude practice surpasses most other practices – it's portable, and you don't even need to buy comfortable clothes, new sneakers, or download an app. And given the chronic conditions of inequality, dramatic political differences, and rancor and anger exploding in the world, it would be worth sticking to a stress relief practice that is quick, easy, and painless. While keeping a gratitude practice is not designated in the literature as a stress relief technique, it will certainly combat the physiological and mental effects of stress on your nervous system, mood, reactions, and relationships, when you practice it daily.

We're not denying our negative feelings or ignoring the political strife or horrors around the world by practicing gratitude on a daily basis. We're acknowledging that our focus can be easily highjacked by a curveball thrown by your boss, a medical diagnosis, or a family squabble. Dealing with sudden bad news at home or at work can quickly obliterate what is good about your neighbor, your health, or the abundance you have in your life.

This book is quite simply for anyone whose blocks get in the way of them genuinely wanting to feel better.

This book is for anyone who needs science to back up a simple self-help practice. It's for anyone who has tried to stick to practices and tools but feels defeated when they fall off the wagon. It's for anyone who doesn't trust that the simple act of gratitude can change almost every aspect of their life.

It's time to do it differently.

If you always do what you've always done, you'll always get what you've always gotten.

My hope is that you use the tools in this book to clear whatever has been blocking you from using this incredible, and incredibly simple, superpower.

My hope is that after clearing your blocks to gratitude, you will feel deeply inspired to start and stick to a consistent gratitude practice.

My hope is that you allow yourself to bring in a gratitude practice that will improve your life in ways you couldn't even imagine right now.

In **Part 1** of this book, I will tell you why practicing gratitude in my life was good in theory, but remained elusive for so many years before it became one of my most cherished self-care practices.

In **Part 2**, I'll explore the emotional, physical, spiritual, and relationship costs of holding onto your blocks. I will discuss the downside of feeling better, and give you the questions you need to ask yourself to get to the bottom of the puzzling self-sabotaging behavior that blocks your success and happiness.

By the time you get to **Part 3**, you'll be ready to learn how to use EFT or Tapping to clear the three major blocks to using a gratitude practice. This tool will help you empty your container of past emotional conflicts, raise your self-esteem so you start valuing yourself and your needs, and identify and eliminate the fears and beliefs that fuel your self-sabotaging behavior. Then the path will be clear for you to be inspired to tap into the superpower of gratitude.

*The results I have seen in myself and
my clients of pairing the clearing tool of EFT with the
superpower of gratitude have been nothing short of miraculous.*

In **Part 4**, I will include **Before and After Stories** from real people who faithfully use a gratitude practice. Their stories will include how their life was unfolding before they started a practice; why, when, and how they incorporate gratitude into their lives; and why they feel inspired to stick to their practices now. In addition, I will include my 7 favorite gratitude practices.

In **Part 5**, I will invite you to start a **30-Day Gratitude Challenge** to change your life for the better.

The solution to clearing your blocks and feeling better is not in a pill bottle, the gym, a new partner, or in your bank account. When you use the tool of EFT to clear your container and free yourself from your past, you'll enjoy the exponentially positive results of feeling emotionally free, and be inspired to conduct your gratitude practices every day.

*Clear your blocks to
tapping into the superpower of gratitude
and you will transform your life.*

Yes, Thank You • 13

How to Use This Book

I recommend reading through this book with an open mind. Drop any misconceptions you have about the practice of gratitude being just a simplistic self-help technique. By the time you get to Part 3, you will have collected enough data to know what blocks you from such a potentially transformational practice. Then, I'll guide you to use EFT to clear the fears, beliefs, and behaviors that are getting in the way of the transformation you deserve.

*Practicing gratitude is
the gift that keeps on giving.*

Available at your fingertips is a free superpower that will amplify your joy and happiness and help you feel better in every area of your life. If you're not tapping into this superpower consistently, let me show you how to remove the blocks and expand your capacity for happiness, joy, and emotional health.

I look forward to supporting you to use the superpower of gratitude to help you *feel better and be better* every day.

To your health, Carol Look

Scan this QR code or go to your *Yes, Thank You* book portal at www.theyescode.com/thankyou for EFT videos and supporting materials for this book.

PART ONE
MY STORY

CHAPTER 1
My Blocks

Throughout my childhood, there was a lot to appreciate about my life. I often felt grateful for my friends, my family, and the educational experiences I enjoyed, but I didn't do anything more with these occasional glimpses of gratitude. Gratitude was an emotion, but so were my feelings of fear, hurt, and sadness about my parents' alcoholism.

After graduating college, and for the first few years of working in a high-stress corporate job in New York, I knew all about the popular habit of gratitude journaling to help you feel better and acknowledge what was good about your life. But I didn't start and keep to a consistent *gratitude practice* until much later. It wasn't that I was actively resisting a practice, I just didn't feel pulled in that direction, or inspired enough to commit to it. I'd like to think that if I had known the impressive research on the positive results, I might have started earlier. But the truth is, I didn't feel drawn towards gratitude as a practice because my emotional container was already too full. I didn't know it at the time, but the space I had in my container was crowded out by the old emotional garbage that had been stored there. *And there was a lot of old garbage.*

I'm telling you my story and why I wasn't practicing gratitude regularly so that you might start to see in yourself what blocks have been in your way. I want you to be able to understand why your emotional capacity for joy and positive energy isn't bigger, and then use the tools I will be providing in Chapter 4 to empty your emotional container of painful material, so you can take advantage of the superpower of practicing gratitude.

If I had known back then what I know now, my life would have been dramatically different – less anxiety, less fear, more hope, more joy, better health, more optimism. But I didn't know what I know now. I have worked on my regret and have forgiven myself for being where I was back then. I was doing the best I could considering that, at times, I was barely keeping my head above water.

So if practicing gratitude is the gift that keeps on giving, why wasn't I practicing it every single day of my life? What limited my container for contentment? Perhaps I could have claimed that I was too busy, but since making a gratitude list takes mere minutes a day, that wasn't a legitimate block to keeping a gratitude practice. The real reason was that my emotional conflicts, low self-esteem, and self-sabotaging behaviors filled my container to its breaking point, dictating the level of success and happiness I had space for, or even thought I deserved.

Emotional conflicts, low self-esteem and self-sabotaging behaviors always run the show.

When I learned that my emotions, low self-esteem, and self-sabotaging behavior were producing all the results I was getting in my life – good and bad – I was able to understand my *why nots* better – why the desire to stick to a gratitude practice would lose out to being busy, worried, stressed out, or unable to tolerate more happiness. I identified the three main blocks that caused me to ignore, forget, or neglect practicing gratitude:

1. I was preoccupied with the chaos and emotional dysfunction in my family; my container was already overflowing with painful emotions. This preoccupation with emotional conflicts led to the second reason I wasn't consistently practicing gratitude.

2. I suffered from low self-esteem and the inevitable self-care neglect that accompanies the belief that you are just not that valuable. Low self-esteem and the habits that it produces led to the third reason my emotional space for contentment was so limited.

3. As a result of my emotional pain and low self-esteem, I was engaged in self-sabotaging behavior – getting in my own way to protect myself from feelings or consequences I feared. I didn't want to stand out, shine, or feel my deep pain, so I used self-sabotage as a way to interfere with my success in my personal and professional life.

Because of these three blocks, I was unaware that the best superpower available to all human beings was literally only one thought away.

Let's unpack these blocks.

Preoccupation

First of all, I was drowning in emotional confusion and pain from my family dysfunction as a result of my parents' alcoholism. For the first few decades of my life, I essentially survived, getting through by focusing on good grades, sports, and great friends in high school and college; and later in my career, by focusing on building professional friendships and connections. I was so preoccupied with the heartache caused by my mother's drinking, then later my father's, that I didn't have any emotional space for a tool such as keeping a gratitude list. My existing container was too full of worry and pain. My focus was on finding a strategy to fix my parents – the impossible dream – *not on helping myself feel better.*

What I knew from watching my mother interact with her friends and family was that being generous, kind, and connecting with people was fun, brought emotional contentment, and created many moments of joy. She was a walking gratitude practice. She expressed her appreciation towards others, and you knew that she didn't take her good life and healthy children for granted. People loved to be around her positive spirit, and she consistently made others feel like they were special. To be the object of her attention was a happy place to be. But she didn't have the tools that we have now, and she didn't know how to empty her container. She struggled with her drinking for her entire adult life, and when she started to drink, she would lose her connection to herself and the source of her gratitude, and once she got started, like most alcoholics, she couldn't or wouldn't stop drinking.

If you read my best-selling book ***The Yes Code***, you'll know that my mother and I were extremely close emotionally, and yet because of her drinking struggles, she broke my heart on a regular basis. Dozens of times. And like an innocent teenager, I would feel hopeful again and again, thinking "this time" she'd stay sober. It would be fair to say that *I fell for it* when she stopped drinking periodically. I was blinded by her resilience when she turned those positive corners. I couldn't predict when she would relapse, and eventually, I'd feel confident she was sticking to her program of sobriety, and I'd let my guard down. Then whammo, out of the blue, she'd start drinking again.

I can't explain the sick feeling that would ooze through my body when I realized she had started drinking. Her repeated relapses, especially when they came after long periods of sobriety, made me feel helpless, hurt, frustrated, and powerless. In addition to feeling sad and upset about her relapses, the pattern left me in a chronic state of apprehension – I was always waiting for the other shoe to drop. This fear and threat from my childhood made me hypervigilant about other people's moods and set me up to look for signs that something was going to go wrong with bosses, jobs, boyfriends, and my health. This pattern of hypervigilance drained my immune system, and of course contributed to my insomnia. My poor nervous system never got a break. It set me up to be highly sensitive to what other people were feeling, regardless of what words were coming out of their mouths. This put my nervous system on a hair trigger, and made me so focused on the energy of other people's moods and feelings that all I cared about was being alert enough to see *it* coming. The "it" could have been someone's mood swing, a relapse, a betrayal, an angry outburst, it didn't really matter. There was only one goal – *to be emotionally safe*.

My mother went in and out of rehabilitation facilities. She sometimes stayed sober for long periods of time, sometimes drank immediately after her release. There were years of uncertainty, heartache, and helplessness – all emotional states that strained my peace of mind and hijacked my focus. And her drinking was all technically a secret – we weren't supposed to talk about it, even though everyone knew about it. I could tell if she had started drinking just by looking at her, before she even opened her mouth to say hello. I could feel it. The alarms would go off instantly, and I'd feel that sick feeling before I could even name the problem.

There was a drunken car ride home from a party once where my mother was weaving all over the tiny back roads in the dark. When I told her friend later, I was told to be quiet about it. There was an accident at school when I was 15, where she smashed our blue station wagon near the carpooling area, but by some stroke of divine intervention, she didn't hit anyone or hurt herself. There were countless arguments that started with me saying, "I know you've been drinking" and ended with her insisting, "Don't be silly, of course I haven't." This wore me down and depleted my energy. Throughout it all, I tried to focus on my friends, sports, and schoolwork, later on my job responsibilities, and further down the road, attending graduate school.

But there was always this dull ache I couldn't quite capture – like a computer program operating in the background – causing doubt and confusion and triggering questions such as: *What else could I do to prevent it?* and *Why wouldn't she stop drinking when we've begged her to stop?* This background mind chatter reminded me of New York City apartments with thin walls where you could always hear the faint sound of your neighbor's music, arguments, or them banging around in the kitchen.

If you haven't lived through a relationship with an alcoholic, this pattern will likely sound odd to you. You may even question how a parent could keep drinking after glaring problems, family arguments, and repeated ruptured trust. Or how loved ones could keep hoping with their fingers crossed when it was clear the alcoholic/addict wasn't willing or able to change. But this is the most prevalent pattern in a family struggling with the disease of alcoholism.

After we staged an intervention, my mother was sent to one of the most well-known treatment facilities in the country. The counselors strongly advised that the family members come for "family week" to support the process of confronting the alcoholic to break down their denial. It was during this family week of treatment that I found my calling to help others. This changed my life for the better, but it was only the start of my new path, and the challenges with my family were far from over.

The pain and heartache weren't constant, but the worrying was always there, as I had learned to look over my shoulder, listen for new sounds, examine facial expressions, or hold my breath so I could hear what my parents were fighting about. Could I ever trust her when she went to the grocery store? Could I ever believe her when she claimed she was "fine"? Could I ever really let down my guard even after long stretches of sobriety? My immune system was a mess, my insomnia was interfering with my functioning at home and at work, and my stress levels were off the charts and wearing me down.

Attending Al-Anon – the 12 step program for family members of alcoholics – and starting therapy after my mother came home from this particular facility definitely helped relieve the emotional pain I was carrying, but it wasn't enough. Yes, I learned that I wasn't alone – way too many people were suffering with the same problems. I learned that someone else's drinking wasn't my fault. That was invaluable. But I didn't suffer from self-blame so much as a deep, and, sadly, misguided desire to find the cause and cure. I wanted to understand why someone would drink, get in trouble, stop, and start drinking again. I was always searching to uncover and fix the circumstances that triggered this cycle.

> ***Of course I couldn't identify someone else's reasons, triggers, or chemistry, but that didn't stop me from trying.***

So even though I had graduated from college and was working in the corporate world, much of my headspace was spent anxiously anticipating my mother's next relapse. *I wasn't thinking of gratitude, I was thinking about the next crisis.*

Again, my emotional preoccupation with a close family member with the diagnosable disease of alcoholism was never off my radar. This focus naturally eclipsed my search for effective healing tools that I could have used to my advantage.

It's worth mentioning that if someone had asked me to practice gratitude when my mother had relapsed, I might have decked them. When you're preoccupied with a frightening and negative situation, you have no more bandwidth and are rarely open to positive suggestions. I have no idea what I would have been able to appreciate at those moments when I felt the jolt upon finding out she had relapsed. That she hadn't driven anywhere that day? That I wasn't living at home anymore? Of course even in difficult times there are always circumstances and blessings to appreciate, *but actively caring for my own well-being wasn't on my list until much later.*

If my container hadn't been so full of emotional turmoil, I sometimes wonder if I would have smoked so addictively, dabbled in harder drugs to relieve my anxiety, or used overeating to quiet my grief. I wasn't handed a gratitude practice when I was anxious, I was handed a joint by a friend.

Later, I wondered if I would have even chosen my first career in the corporate world if I had known how to take care of myself. I wonder if I would have been so unaware of the cumulative effects of stress that my work and the situations I put myself in stored in my body. If my container hadn't been so full of pain, I might have been able to reap the benefits of a gratitude practice at an early age.

There were many moments in my life where I look back now and realize that if someone had invited me to express my gratitude during an emotionally painful period, I would have been unable to see the value, and therefore, would have dismissed it. My solitary desire was to help my mother, not focus on how to improve my own life, health, and well-being.

Over time, I matured, sought more help, and reduced the amount of time I spent preoccupied with trying to change my parents. But whenever my mother relapsed, it was always a stab in the heart. So, while my preoccupation decreased dramatically over time, my underlying grief was always dormant, waiting to be revived. This blocked my ability to search for more contentment and peace, as I didn't even know it was possible to feel dramatically better. Under these conditions, my container had little room for joy, let alone positive self-care. So essentially, I learned the lesson that I couldn't afford the luxury of self-care because I needed to look for signs of threat and danger around every corner.

Low Self-Esteem

My second block to keeping a gratitude practice was that being raised by parents who were genuinely loving but who often chose alcohol over me created confusion, frustration, and helplessness. I didn't understand that I was valuable, or when I did, it was quickly negated by an upsetting drinking episode or my father's temper. I could detail a million times when my parents expressed their love, interest, and appreciation of us, but when they drank anyway, I didn't feel *deserving* of that value. My self-esteem was low enough that it didn't occur to me to invest in myself – unconsciously I was convinced I didn't deserve it. The classic advice from twelve step programs and counseling recommended you put yourself first and stop trying to save your alcoholic. But that doesn't sink in very easily as good advice until you're sick and tired of chasing solutions that would inevitably dissolve with the next relapse.

I didn't really pivot emotionally until I had gotten my hopes up for the millionth time, only to have them dashed an equal number of times. Until repeated health crises brought me to my emotional and physical knees, I wasn't even aware that my low self-esteem was undermining my self-care. I was basically asleep at the wheel.

Neglecting my self-care ended up stressing my immune system and contributing to my physical ailments. As you may have read in **The Yes Code**, throughout the late 1980s and 1990s, I suffered from multiple cysts, a breast tumor, a polyp in my throat, and a globular hemangioma in my hand. All of these abnormal growths needed to be removed with a scalpel and other tools that make me dizzy when I think about them. And yet I continued to burn the candle at both ends, first in the corporate world and then in graduate school. I didn't get enough sleep, stayed out too late, worried too much, and got away with not taking care of my physiological and emotional needs for years. Eventually, I stopped being able to recover so quickly, and started listening to the signals my body was offering.

With time, therapy, and support groups, I eventually started taking better care of myself. Since I was generally satisfied in my job, successful in my friendships, and happy in my marriage, my weakened immune system and general anxiety largely went unnoticed. My yo-yo-ing weight, mystery tumors, and debilitating insomnia mirrored my stress levels, but didn't send out a big enough SOS for anyone to notice. After years of feeling defeated by a recurring fever, I finally felt motivated to make regular changes to caring for myself and my well-being.

If you have low self-esteem, you won't truly believe that you *deserve that much happiness*. However, I didn't know it was one of my challenges back then. What I know now is that people with low self-esteem don't take very good care of themselves. They have trouble feeling worthy, can't say no, and they struggle to create good boundaries. When you suffer from low self-esteem, you don't value your needs or feelings that much. Unlike the airplane advice about putting the oxygen mask on yourself first, people with low self-esteem rarely make themselves a priority. So, in hindsight it's obvious that I didn't feel deserving of more joy, contentment, and happiness. Some of my boyfriends were trainwrecks, my eating habits were atrocious, and working too hard after graduate school was a given – all symptoms of low self-esteem and not feeling worthy of more self-care. Back then, I was just doing what I always did – surviving fairly well while not showing enough outer pain to attract attention. I was extremely high functioning, so it didn't look like I was drowning from the excruciating inner pain that drove my feelings, beliefs, and behavior.

Unlike an actual death, a loved one's repeated alcoholic relapses trigger grief in a different way. While this sounds dramatic, it felt like I lost my mother over and over again. Just as I'd start to relax, she'd relapse, and I'd learn the lessons *don't get your hopes up* and *don't let your guard down*. Both seemed like foolish ideas. It left me trying to build a shell of protection with emotional glue and duct tape that would inevitably deteriorate when I felt my mother's genuine remorse. Her regret and insistence that it would never happen again made my heart melt, and my feeble boundaries would collapse.

In college and in my first job in the financial industry, I didn't know building self-esteem was an inside job. I only knew what felt normal – looking outside of myself to feel better. Whether the vehicle to feeling better was a new boyfriend, exciting substances, a bigger paycheck, or work success, these outside goodies never stuck to my ribs. They were empty calories and did even more damage as they left my system.

My journey of improving and rebuilding my self-esteem enough to make my self-care a priority wasn't a linear progression, and yours won't be either. I had many starts and stops along the way. In boarding school, I had wonderful friendships, and intellectual and emotional growth spurts that were age appropriate. But I'd call home and find out that my mother was drinking and couldn't come to the phone. My mood would deteriorate for hours. I'd feel forlorn and helpless all over again. In college I'd call home and hear in her voice that she had relapsed, and my mood would sink like a stone tossed into the middle of a pond.

Self-Sabotaging Behavior

The third reason I wasn't practicing gratitude on a regular basis was that I was engaged in self-sabotaging behavior that blocked me from even wanting to be at my best. The positive intent of self-sabotaging behavior is to keep yourself safe from emotional risk or pain. I smoked and ate to obliterate my emotional pain, I procrastinated to protect myself from standing out, and my perfectionism stopped me from being judged and criticized so much, or so I thought. I tried to keep a lid on my professional success because I didn't want to stand out and be the target of anyone's jealousy or envy. I didn't want to feel my pain, so I smoked everything I could get my hands on and repeatedly gained and lost the same 20-25 pounds. The self-sabotaging behavior kept me playing small – an attempt to keep myself safe.

So, it was the perfect storm. I was preoccupied by my mother's drinking habits and the pain they caused; I had low self-esteem, and as a result, behaved as if I didn't deserve to take care of myself; and my self-sabotaging behavior kept a lid on my success. These blocks all created chronic stress, sucking any remaining oxygen out of what was left in my container. There was simply no room to explore new techniques for expanding my joy and contentment.

I hadn't yet been introduced to the breakthrough tool of EFT Tapping to clear the blocks to expanding my emotional capacity for happiness. Talk therapy and Al-Anon weren't enough. Expressing challenging emotional conflicts and hearing other people talk about struggling with an alcoholic at home temporarily took the edge off my anxiety. But my container for joy was still too full of pain, and that meant I was still in the dark.

I was moving as fast as I could, but that shoe was always about to drop – at work, at home, and in my health. I was enjoying my work tremendously, taking advantage of the New York night life and important friendships, but I wasn't actively seeking more contentment and joy. I seemed genuinely happy to anyone who knew me. The stress seemed normal to me, and I was an expert at trying to manage it. My agitated nervous system and the difficulty I had calming my anxiety was what I had always known so I wasn't looking for any new techniques and tools. This left little room or motivation for searching for a practice such as gratitude.

Over the years, I steadily emptied my container of painful emotions, improved my self-esteem by identifying and taking care of my needs more, and started to clear the real reasons I was sabotaging my success. I was a successful counselor, had completed my doctoral degree in clinical hypnosis, was happily married, generally content, and in good health (besides my tumors and fluctuating weight), but I was still struggling with some of my blocks. It wasn't until I learned about the weird new therapy called EFT Tapping, and began using it to release old traumas, fears, and limiting beliefs, that I felt an internal spark and recognized that there could be so much more for me. Like the first sounds of the popcorn kernels waking up in the microwave bag, I started to come alive.

I was fascinated by the EFT concept – tapping on acupuncture points to calm down the brain – and applied for the trainings as my schedule would allow. Embarking upon my Tapping career would soon help me support my clients, stand up for myself, set strong boundaries, and take better care of my health. I stopped holding my breath, waiting for the next crisis, and started expanding my capacity for joy and peace.

Progress

Once I learned about the power of EFT in 1997, I started experimenting with using Tapping with my clients in my private practice. I, and they, had immediate shifts in behaviors and a noticeable reduction in their anxiety and stress levels. Because I was a hypnotist, I was exclusively referred clients for anxiety relief, smoking cessation, and weight loss. I offered them Tapping in addition to hypnosis. Clients would come back to their follow-up session after learning Tapping exercises and they would say, *What did you do?* They noticed decreased cravings, less anxiety, lower stress levels, and their hope for finally healing long-standing traumatic cycles increased. While I was focused on offering this new tool to my clients, *my insomnia disappeared*. This was truly a game changer for my physical and emotional well-being.

I continued to use Tapping on myself and my clients, with three dramatic benefits: (1) I was able to dilute the amount of time spent worried or upset about family issues; I healed many old wounds and unhealthy behavior patterns related to growing up with alcoholism, making more room for joy in my container; (2) I released the heavy emotional weight of events and beliefs that contributed to my low self-esteem and feeling unworthy; and (3) I was able to recognize and heal the underlying need to sabotage myself. This healing process enabled me to hold more success, happiness, and peace of mind, no matter what was going on with my family.

I felt considerably better after using Tapping on my own childhood issues, which, in turn, made me feel more deserving of joy. This was the turning point for me in my personal journey – I used Tapping to quiet enough of the emotional distress and noise, and as a result, had more emotional space to be curious and drawn to other tools such as a gratitude practice. If you need a case study, I am exhibit A. I reaped enormous benefits from the Tapping practice to make space for me to want to expand my capacity for emotional freedom, including being inspired to use a gratitude practice.

I had started hearing more about people using a gratitude practice as a way to "manifest" material goodies in their lives. (This was many years before the movie *The Secret* came out.) So, I started getting more interested in using gratitude as a means of manifesting financial success. I had made a vow that after growing up hearing constant arguments between my parents about financial trouble, I wasn't going to live that way. I was committed to finding a path to financial freedom. I was seduced into expressing gratitude for this shallow, materialistic reason, but I stuck with it because it simply made me feel better, more hopeful, and more aligned with my purpose in life. **My why was finally getting bigger than my why not.**

By 2003, my *why nots* (blocks) had been reduced enough that my *why* was leading the way. I was using a gratitude practice regularly, experimenting and playing with my new game. I was reciting gratitude lists, expressing gratitude on my morning walks, and focusing on creative ways to express appreciation. Within a couple of days of starting my new practice, Gary Craig, the creator of EFT, asked me to teach a workshop with him following one of his basic beginners' classes. He would gather the audience, hire the videographer, and hand the audience over to me after his introductory day on EFT. We decided I would teach on the topic of *Attracting Abundance with EFT*, which later became the title of my first book.

Over the next few days, the significance of this invitation began to dawn on me. He trusted me enough to put his sold-out audience in my hands. He had never asked anyone else to teach in conjunction with him, nor provided such an amazing opportunity. Whether it was a simple coincidence or not, I connected this opportunity to my new-found gratitude practice. While exhilarating, it also spooked me a little. Was expressing gratitude really this powerful? Was it this easy to improve your life, receive extraordinary invitations, gain more financial freedom and "stuff" that you wanted? This opportunity put me on the map as a go-to trusted EFT expert, which has shaped the rest of my career to this day.

Around the same time period when I was experimenting with expressing gratitude, I would turn down the volume on my answering machine daily so I could carve out some quiet time for this new practice, write out my list, and count my blessings. One morning, during one of these 10-minute time periods, a former client from California left a message saying she had finally gathered the money to pay me for a bounced check (for which her replacement check had also bounced) and that I would be receiving $1,500 in the mail. I had already written off this loss with my accountant, so I wasn't expecting to hear from her or ever see this money again. This time, the timing was too close (the same 10-minute period) to write off as a coincidence. Again, while I was dabbling in the "manifestation" arena, I couldn't deny these positive results. More importantly, I couldn't discount how good focusing on gratitude made me feel.

Experiencing positive benefits from a regular gratitude practice wouldn't have been possible for me if I hadn't used Tapping consistently to remove the blocks I had to feeling deserving of more peace and joy. Using EFT regularly helped me let go of long-held painful emotions and negative beliefs about what I deserved, released layers of anxiety and grief, eliminated frustrations and helplessness, and erased the real reasons I was keeping a lid on my personal and professional success. My insomnia had dissolved, I was more confident and relaxed, I learned to set and keep strong boundaries, and my second career was taking off.

*I finally had more room for gratitude
and for the hope and contentment it provided.*

Eventually I created a branch of EFT called "Gratitude Tapping" that many practitioners have adopted. I have also incorporated many gratitude practices into my self-care routine, and feel the benefits deeply. Now, no matter what is going on in my professional arena, family life, or in the chaotic outside world, I can reach for my tools and immediately feel more peaceful, secure, and more emotionally free on the spot.

After working on myself with EFT Tapping and changing the underlying anxiety quite quickly, I ran into two additional and surprising reasons for self-sabotaging myself that limited my capacity for enjoying the benefits of gratitude. These two additional blocks could have led me to sabotage my career and happiness. They tempted me to play small and shrink my container for joy. Staying under the radar would have solved the "problems" I was confronted with, but would have made me miserable.

The first unexpected block I bumped into was feeling guilty about my exploding professional success. As I watched colleagues get stuck, or family members get sick, my success created internal emotional tension and guilt about my own progress.

At an EFT workshop I attended, I had an opportunity to have a session with EFT Creator, Gary Craig, with me as the client. I don't remember what he asked me, but the crux of the session was my guilt. As my career was taking off and I was genuinely more content and happier than I'd been in a long time, my younger sister was dying of breast cancer. I described my guilt to him. I don't remember what we tapped on exactly, but it obviously worked, because my guilt diminished enough that I didn't hold myself back professionally or personally.

My sister died about 6 months later, leaving a shattered husband, kids, parents, siblings, and friends. I grieved with them all, wholeheartedly, publicly and privately, and yet I was also able to continue to move forward with my passion for helping others.

The second unexpected block was my being perplexed and upset by other people's reactions to my success. I noticed that as I released some old hurt and pain, I felt better and more confident, and my professional success started to explode. As my professional success increased, I became aware of other people's negative reactions to my success. Gary Craig putting me on the EFT map triggered other people's jealousy and envy.

I noticed colleagues saying snarky comments about my success. I was younger than many of the practitioners who were in the Tapping field – long time psychotherapists who had discovered EFT around the same time I had. They were clearly envious of my relationship with Gary, noticed the opportunities he gave me, and found small-minded ways of knocking me down. This was an invitation to continue working on *my reactions to their reactions*. I tapped on my guilt, my fear of their responses, and my hurt at their suggestions that I shouldn't be in the spotlight. I expressed gratitude daily for all my gifts and all these challenges. I neutralized my fear of their reactions so that instead of feeling compelled to play small, I continued to excel in my work. This allowed me to continue to use a consistent gratitude practice and enjoy the benefits of calming me down, taking better care of myself, and expanding my capacity for joy.

As I said earlier, my path to practicing gratitude wasn't linear. But once I started using EFT to heal my old wounds and release the intense anxiety in my nervous system, I was able to clean out and dispose of old emotional files that were crammed in my container. This allowed me to expand my desire and capacity for joy, happiness, and contentment. Once I cleaned out and made space in my emotional container, I was able to see how I was hurting myself with low self-esteem behavior such as not standing up for myself; and self-sabotaging behaviors such as procrastination, perfectionism, and avoiding my deep emotional conflicts. And as a result, I was able to release the chronic stress that accompanied these three blocks and make use of more tools that amplified positive benefits.

In hindsight, it's very clear what kept me from starting a gratitude practice earlier in my life: the preoccupation with my emotional pain; my low self-esteem which told me that I didn't deserve more joy; and using self-sabotaging behavior in an attempt to keep myself playing small and safe. In turn, these challenges created a perfect landscape for me to ignore the benefits of a superpower such as practicing gratitude.

> *I discovered that I was actually*
> *afraid to be happier,*
> *because it would take my guard down.*

I just couldn't hold or absorb that much optimism or contentment when I was always afraid the other shoe would drop. I wasn't actually trying to feel happier; I was looking to help my mother stop drinking, and when I finally got the message that I had nothing to do with her drinking, I was just looking for ways to stop feeling my own grief.

As I've detailed, I suffered from anxiety, addictive behavior, and intense grief for many years. And yet not once did a counselor suggest I try a gratitude practice. I talked endlessly in traditional therapy until I finally found EFT which helped me release the negative patterns and old traumas from my nervous system.

Tapping changed my life by releasing my anxiety enough to heal the habit of my insomnia. It supported me in letting go of decades of grief so I could finally lose the extra 25 pounds and keep them off. Tapping helped me increase my income five-fold and more, deepened my capacity to be a good therapist, and strengthened all my relationships, both personal and professional. While it never helped me stop my mother's drinking, and to this day doesn't help me stop my sister's spiraling alcoholic decline, it helped my mood, attitude, and outlook. It took Tapping and healing my emotional conflicts to clear enough space for me to avail myself of the superpower of expressing gratitude.

For years, my students from all over the world have written me detailing the benefits they have found from using EFT Tapping for themselves and with others. The benefits showed up in their health, their self-esteem, their business's bottom line, and in their interactions with their friends and family members.

I continued to work with clients and helped them move from being stuck to feeling free, from feeling insecure to exuding confidence, from clinging to addictive patterns to releasing their compulsions to eat, drink, and smoke to excess. I have taught workshops in all the corners of the world, have treated clients from the ages of 6 to 86, and have heard the same feedback every place I went – *where has this amazing Tapping tool been all my life?*

Without Tapping to clear my emotional blocks, I would never have been able to take advantage of all the myriad benefits of expressing gratitude. Due to the nature of self-sabotage and the habit of getting in my own way, just knowing about the extensive benefits of expressing real and genuine gratitude would not have inspired me to keep a steady or daily practice. I was, after all, still struggling with a container that was already filled to the brim with emotional challenges and facing loss after loss.

Immediately after the attacks of 9-11, I was overwhelmed with many competing emotions of terror and confusion. It didn't occur to me to start a gratitude practice then.

Three months after 9-11, when my younger sister died of metastatic breast cancer – was this a time for someone to suggest I start a gratitude practice? I'm sure I would have ignored the suggestion.

When I was generally feeling low and powerless because of my mother's chronic relapses, I highly doubt that I would have felt enthusiastic about starting a gratitude journal.

And when my mother died suddenly while getting dressed for my father's funeral, that was not the time to practice gratitude, *or so I thought back then.*

You may be in crisis right now, and if I were to tell you this is an ideal time to start a gratitude practice, you might feel angry and frustrated that I wasn't understanding your feelings. I get it. But if you had already been actively clearing your blocks with EFT, and subsequently embracing a gratitude practice, then using it during your most challenging emotional times could be comforting and would speed your healing process. So, while I didn't practice gratitude during these painful times, *I wish I had.* It would have provided me with a deeper perspective, a connection to all the positive aspects about my relationships, and helped heal the grief. It would have provided me with momentary glimpses of light and lifted me out of the darkness.

My wish for you, is that even if you're in crisis, you can both use the tool of EFT to release emotional pain, and start expressing gratitude to find the pockets of joy in your life, even if they've been momentarily eclipsed by grief, hardship, or trauma. There's a famous expression in 12 step programs: *"There are two best times to go to a meeting – when you want to and when you don't want to."* And I think that applies to using a super tool such as EFT and using the superpower of expressing gratitude. Incorporate the habits into your life and then you'll naturally reach for a tool like EFT and automatically use a gratitude practice whether the sun's out or there's a blizzard.

> **You may not believe me and may even be confused by my suggestion, but IT'S ALWAYS A GOOD TIME to count your blessings and express gratitude.**

Even if you're smack in the middle of a life crisis – you've received a diagnosis, you've just lost a pet or a loved one, you've just been handed a pink slip – there are immediate benefits to practicing gratitude. Expressing gratitude doesn't mean you're in denial and it doesn't dismiss the gravity of your crisis, but it is an opportunity to turn your attention to the good in your life and experience small moments of relief available to you.

Because of the blocks I outlined in my life, I literally couldn't take advantage of the many different types of gratitude practices available because my container for emotional success and happiness was already too full and spilling over with pain. It was not until I used EFT to decrease my preoccupation with the family dysfunction, improve my self-esteem, and identify the real reasons I was sabotaging myself, that I was able to "hear" the invitation to use gratitude. My mood, attitude, and life have never been the same.

I still believe in the power of emotional growth through compassionate talk therapy, but the research shows that traumatic experiences get trapped in our physiology and our nervous system, and no amount of talking will dissolve the painful imprints. I needed a body-based energy technology such as EFT Tapping to get out of my downward spiral.

My hope for you is that you identify what blocks have been in your way, so you can use the tools and exercises in Part 3 of this book to release your emotional conflicts and limiting beliefs, make more space in your container, and expand your capacity to cherish your practice of gratitude. Not just because it will make you sleep better, improve your immune system, or lower your risk of hypertension, *but because you deserve to feel better every day of your life.*

When you have more energy and feel better, you have more access to joy and wonder, and when you increase your capacity for joy and wonder, you lower your negative reactions to other people's behavior. And as you lower your reactivity to other people, you expand your capacity to be emotionally present, which makes you a better friend, a more dependable colleague, and a more emotionally grounded family member. Your deeper relaxation will amplify your emotional equanimity and your capacity to be quiet, still, and present.

The high-powered benefits of combining Tapping to clear the emotional blocks with starting a gratitude practice to appreciate the good in your life become exponential – I've seen this unfold in my clients and I'm living proof of the results.

Once you feel emotionally lighter, more settled, and peaceful as a result of releasing the old baggage of fear and trauma, reversing your low self-esteem, and releasing the need to sabotage yourself, then you'll be more open to expressing gratitude, which will improve your sense of optimism, enable you to be a better listener, and contribute to more robust health.

> **YOU DESERVE *the exponential results you can get from releasing the pain with EFT and increasing your joy with gratitude.***

My hope for you is that you will enjoy the astonishing power of EFT Tapping to expand your capacity to feel more joy so you will erase any blocks you might have had to deserving to feel better. This will, in turn, cement your feeling of worthiness and open yourself to experience the superpower of gratitude in your life.

It doesn't matter if, like me, you have been attracted to unsuitable partners, carried extra weight, or cringed when you thought of some of your past behaviors. Finding EFT and clearing my blocks paved the way to utilizing the superpower of gratitude and changed the trajectory of my personal and professional life. Every time I think about the path I was destined to take, it gives me hope. And when I think of being given the honor of empowering another person with these tools, my hope is irrepressible.

I couldn't change my past, but I could transform the pain and heartache, feel better in my present life, and create a more joyful future.

I invite you to hop on this path the first chance you get. Use EFT to release past pain that's clogging your emotional container, raise your self-esteem so you put yourself first more often, and delete the need to sabotage your success. This will expand your desire for more joy and emotional freedom so you can take advantage of gratitude as a superpower. With this expanded capacity for peace, you will reach for more joy, and create a future you can anticipate with pleasure.

In the next part of this book, I will be laying the groundwork to understand the costs of holding onto emotional pain, neglecting our self-care, and scrambling to find ways to sabotage ourselves. This will set the table for Part 3 where I will teach you how to release the blocks to expanding your capacity for more emotional freedom, joy, and happiness. Then you'll be ready for Part 4 where we will explore gratitude stories from people who've worked tirelessly to clear their blocks, and outline gratitude practices I have found most useful. Finally, in Part 5, I will invite you to embark upon my 30-Day Gratitude Challenge to take advantage of this incredible habit and start seeing the results in your life right away.

PART TWO
THE PROBLEM

CHAPTER 2

The Costs

Before we jump into the solution in Part 3, I'm going to unpack the situation that keeps you stuck and unable to engage with gratitude. In my 30 plus years as a psychotherapist, I have found that most people have the same blocks I had, and these obstacles carry tremendous costs – they create chronic stress, and deplete your emotional and physical resources. These chapters will prepare you for Part 3 where I'll teach you how to use an exceptional emotional technology – the super tool of EFT Tapping – to release your blocks and pave the way for engaging with gratitude more fully and consistently.

Let's recap our blocks.

1. <u>Your Container Is Full</u>: Your emotional container is full of unresolved emotional challenges from your past. It's packed with memories of upsetting events, feelings of resentment, guilt, anxiety, fear, and betrayal. Re-living, avoiding, or even repressing these old memories creates chronic stress in your body and your life. Your container is overflowing with your past, so there's no room to embrace the fulfillment that engaging with a consistent gratitude practice could bring you in your present life. It's not your fault that your container is bursting at the seams, but once you know that this is a primary block to feeling better, and that there are reliable tools available for support and healing, you can systematically empty your container, release the stress its contents has created, and then make room for the benefits of a gratitude practice.

2. <u>Low Self-Esteem</u>: Because of these past painful memories and experiences that are stuck in your container, your self-esteem – *how you*

treat yourself and let others treat you – is likely quite low. That means taking care of your needs and your well-being are not at the top of your list. If you were taught to believe that you're just not that valuable, you will not take care of yourself and will have difficulty setting strong boundaries in all your relationships. If you were taught not to value yourself, you also might feel guilty saying no to friends and colleagues, and generally put others first at great expense to yourself. Unfortunately, if you have low self-esteem, you'll behave in ways that perpetuate the feeling of not deserving what you want in your life, which in turn creates a great deal of stress.

3. <u>Self-Sabotaging Behavior</u>: Behaviors such as procrastination, perfectionism, addictions, and creating relationship drama are all examples of getting in your own way so that you don't move forward in your personal or professional life. The positive intent of self-sabotaging behavior is to protect and keep yourself emotionally safe from something you fear – standing out, being visible, or being successful. You're actually using self-sabotaging behavior for a good reason, but it hurts you and impedes your progress at work and at home, creating tremendous pressure and strain in your life.

The chronic stress from these three blocks drains your emotional and physical resources, and as a result, yo*u become less resilient, and more easily triggered.* These reactions make you more vulnerable to becoming emotionally ungrounded and interpersonally irritable. Our focus and attention are easily hijacked by horrific breaking news, and we forget to check if there are any positive events occurring in our own backyard. We argue with someone on the other side of our political viewpoint, become stuck in our opinions, and abandon our humanity. We become addicted to drama at home and at work, and we drain our immune systems with what we eat and drink, and how we sleep. The result is that we are physically depleted and emotionally fragile. It becomes a vicious cycle. Add to that the feeling of being disconnected from our intuition and the inner wisdom available to us, and we are left running on empty, and poorly equipped to handle the demands of our families, jobs, and health.

If you're caught in a cycle of draining your energy because of old painful memories constantly replaying in a loop, treating yourself poorly due to your low self-esteem, and maintaining self-sabotaging patterns in your daily life, you are unlikely to reach for better tools to take care of yourself, much less take advantage of the gifts the superpower of expressing gratitude can give you.

I'm not saying it is easy to turn this situation around. I'm saying that if you don't address these aspects of your current situation, the costs will be exorbitant and will show up emotionally, physically, spiritually, and in your relationships.

Let's examine the costs of each of these primary blocks.

Emotional Costs

The emotional costs of not clearing your past pain, conflicts, and burdens out of your container can be overwhelming. If emotional burdens that occurred upstream in your childhood weren't managed effectively, the downstream fallout will be devastating. They may seem small at first, but then they build into a tidal wave that can overtake your entire system. You'll see the fallout in your relationships at work and at home, you'll notice unmanageable mood swings and reactivity, and unpleasant symptoms will show up in your body. If you're not aware of your emotional state – anxious vs. calm, happy vs. disgruntled, resentful vs. content – then you're not going to be aware of how much your container is overflowing with negativity. When we're not aware, we just keep doing what we've always done, and we don't make the commitment to produce the necessary changes to take care of ourselves.

If you have a container full of unresolved grief, it will eventually show up externally in your life. You might shy away from relationships, use food or drugs to anesthetize the grief, or be unable to handle other people's emotions when they experience losses. If you have a container full of unresolved resentment or anxiety, the unhappiness and weight of these childhood conflicts will create unrest in your adulthood - mood swings, depression, anxiety, and chronic emotional tension. All of these emotional costs lead to disruptions in your ability to relate to your boss, colleagues, children, and partners. When you are suffering from these emotional cycles, it's not easy to search for tools to better your life, and you certainly wouldn't start a gratitude practice. You might even think you're *fine* because you're doing well enough. Dinner is on the table, and you get to work on time, but that's a low bar if you want to improve your levels of contentment and fulfillment.

Many people aren't aware of the negative emotional costs of having a full container. They feel "normal" because they're accustomed to how it feels. It often takes a challenging event in adulthood that triggers an emotional reaction to show the outside world that the person is in trouble emotionally. They have their first panic attack, their drinking becomes out of control, the stress causes overreactive responses at work or at home, and it becomes obvious to others that you are not managing your emotions. If you are aware of the negative costs, you can change your behavior and your results. If you're not aware of the costs, then you'll keep doing what you've always done, and keep missing out on what you deserve – an expanded capacity for happiness, joy, and contentment. Emptying your container from past traumas and emotions means you'll have more presence of mind, feel calmer and less reactive, and be better able to handle the fast balls that life is whizzing by your head.

Sometimes our physicians or health care providers notice our increased anxiety or our tendencies to fall into a depressive slump in the winter. Often our family members notice our increased irritability, or our unnecessary impatience with the kids, even when we don't. As the old expression says, *you can't read the label from inside the jar!*

I know my stress levels have reached a negative tipping point when simple little frustrations trigger an overreaction. I spill my coffee and yell multiple swear words – a reaction that is out of proportion with what happened. My anxiety and stress levels show up in my digestion and sleep habits too, so I get signals from my body informing me when I am out of balance. I also have loving counselors, friends, and family members who recognize when my mood is out of line, and they're willing to share their concerns and invite me to consider what needs my attention.

Notice if you're overreacting or barking at the kids too much. Notice if you're feeling irritable because you are or feel underappreciated by your boss or spouse. Notice if you're emotionally short in interactions with a loved one who doesn't deserve your curtness. These are signs that you need more work on emptying your container. Cars have sensors that tell you when another driver is too close, when passing is unsafe, or when you're slipping in the snow or ice. We need these sensors too.

Once you become aware that you feel out of balance, then you can consciously choose to get support. Noticing that your emotional reactions are too "hot" is the first step to feeling motivated – then inspired – to start new habits and make lifestyle changes. You can consciously choose to ask for support to empty your container.

Physical Costs

The physical costs of not emptying your container, not improving your self-esteem, and continuing the patterns of self-sabotaging behaviors are often more obvious than the emotional costs. When you are exhausted, gain weight, or get a diagnosis related to excessive stress, it's written in bold letters all over you: *Look at me, I'm not taking good care of myself.* Your doctor may even warn you against the late nights at work, advise you to lay off sugar and alcohol, or prescribe a vacation to alleviate your disgruntled mood. When you feel better, you'll start to take better care of yourself.

If your container is too full of old memories and upsets, then there's a chronic drain on your physiology through your nervous system. You may get more viruses every year, may develop sleep problems, may gain weight, or use substances to try and calm yourself down. Then you'll have to deal with the consequences of trying to manage your stress. When your self-esteem is low, you tend to run yourself into the ground physically. The neighbor's request for a favor comes before your need for a meal or for sleep. When the boss asks for one more assignment, you say yes even though you're at your breaking point. When you keep sabotaging yourself, you will drain your resources and feel physically depleted, as if you have one foot on the brake and one foot on the gas.

So, in addition to juggling the blocks of a full container, low self-esteem, and self-sabotaging behavior, you'll struggle with the physical repercussions of carrying these blocks. When you start to take better care of yourself, you often feel compelled to engage in self-care practices more often – you start protecting your sleep, guarding your energy, and unhooking from people who drain your resources. When you make your physical health a priority, your life will change, but it can take some time to get there. It took me several diagnoses, 3 unrelated tumors, and a chronic infection before I got the message to slow down and pay attention to what was draining my energy. *Just because I could live on very little sleep, doesn't mean I should have.*

When you feel exhausted or drained, you don't reach for healthier behaviors or practices to help yourself. You literally don't have enough energy for anything but getting through the day. You ignore important warning signals from your body and engage in lazy habits like grabbing a quick unhealthy lunch at your desk that further degrade your physical stamina and resiliency. It's a very unhealthy cycle.

It wasn't until I had made significant progress with moving my blocks that I was finally able to engage more with tools to help myself. I started a meditation practice and discovered the value of gratitude. Before that time, I was treading water frantically, but not getting anywhere. And there was so much emotional noise, I didn't have any room for anything else. My hands were full, and all of my attention was being paid to the various fears I was juggling. If you feel exhausted, run down, overwhelmed, underappreciated, or preoccupied, you won't listen to the signals telling you that it's time to slow down, much less reach for gratitude, no matter how much of a superpower it is.

A primary physical response to not clearing your blocks is feeling generally run down by life and its stressors. Unfortunately, these physical symptoms start to erode your physical health at even deeper levels – you don't just feel tired or lacking energy, you might start struggling with intense insomnia, serious hypertension, mystery symptoms that eventually lead to auto-immune disorders, or an emergency visit to a doctor where you'll be ordered to change your lifestyle habits. Don't wait for a serious diagnosis before you start clearing your blocks and taking better care of yourself.

Relationship Costs

The cost of not managing your primary blocks is very expensive to your relationships and show up as intimacy issues, communication challenges, and an inability to connect with others in genuine and authentic ways. These blocks take up a lot of space and battery power, and leave you with low energy and a reluctance to have difficult but necessary conversations. Not clearing these blocks will also make you quick to overreact, and unable to hear your partner, friends, or colleagues. Many couples report that they feel distant or out of touch, even though they live together. They have often stopped communicating emotionally, and are engaged in a transactional relationship. Dialogue such as "You pick up the kids after soccer, and I'll make dinner," becomes the primary interaction.

Discord in any relationship is a sign to stop, slow down, and examine your priorities. Maybe you're feeling the effects of these blocks with a colleague at work, or with an old friend. It might be time to examine your self-esteem issues, or examine whether your childhood reactions are interfering with your adult intimacy, your communication style, or your ability to show empathy. Once you start paying attention to feelings of discord in any of your relationships, you start noticing when your resentment is building and when you feel under-appreciated. You can then initiate conversations where you communicate more clearly, respectfully, and intimately.

Spiritual Costs

The spiritual cost of not clearing your blocks shows up as not having the space or interest to pursue a spiritual life. You might feel an emotional flatness or a sense of disconnection from something greater than yourself. If you're not interested in pursuing a relationship with a spiritual aspect to life, that's fine too. But when you're struggling to just get by, spiritual comfort will be out of reach. Most people recognize that feeling resentful, overwhelmed, irritable, or impatient will dull their connection with a higher power, spirit, divine intelligence, or whatever you relate to as the force that's keeping the planets in motion.

Yuberka

Yuberka is a 49-year-old woman from The Dominican Republic. She is the right-hand assistant to a famous hair stylist in New York. She told me that she used to be connected to gratitude when she was a child, but lost this connection over the years while navigating a troubled marriage, raising 2 children, and managing difficult personalities on a variety of jobs. She felt she had become disconnected from this powerful emotion, and felt almost dead inside.

After using Tapping to embrace the emotions she had been neglecting, she felt calmer, was able to focus on her priorities, and take care of her own needs. This, in turn, allowed her to resume her daily habit of expressing gratitude. She said she reconnected to God through nature – her spiritual source – and found life to be easier, sweeter, and simpler to manage. She said she is often moved to tears when she tunes in to her feelings of gratitude and appreciation. This has also reconnected her to her emotional center and her purpose in life.

Yuberka's story is one of the thousands I have heard showing the emotional, physical, spiritual, and relationship costs of maintaining these negative but familiar cycles caused by our primary blocks. They can cost us emotional peace and calm, healthy communication, immune system strength, relationship satisfaction, and even shorten our life expectancy. In addition, these blocks blind us to the value of self-care tools: chief among them, the superpower of practicing gratitude.

The research also indicates that the practice of expressing gratitude is a complete game changer when it comes to our stress response and the biological consequences of being chronically hypervigilant in our lives. The findings all point to the probability of feeling significantly better in our personal and professional lives if we practice expressing gratitude regularly. *If...that's the key word here.*

The first step to clearing our blocks is being aware of how and where we're struggling. Once we know this, we can become aware of the expensive repercussions in our lives. The blocks and their costs are extremely hard on our nervous systems, so we need to clear them and evaluate what issues need our focus and commitment, or what parts of our lives deserve attention and a reboot.

The Good News

Once you become aware of your current situation and all the costs associated with your blocks, you can get to work on healing and changing the outdated and expensive patterns. The solution is to empty out your container of past hurts and traumas; reverse the patterns of low self-esteem by engaging in daily acts that allow you to value yourself; and uncover and clear the real reasons you feel the need to sabotage your success and happiness. After using the right tools, these improvements will set the stage for starting and sticking to a gratitude practice. You'll be able to enjoy the incredible benefits detailed by the research studies about the superpower of gratitude and feel more alive and fulfilled in your life.

You may have started to take care of yourself, but then stopped because of the blocks. You may have been so overwhelmed that you couldn't even think of starting or keeping up a gratitude practice. The difference this time is that *you know why.*

You know now that your self-protective instincts kicked in before and stopped you from taking care of yourself. You know that your past overwhelmed you. You know that you didn't feel worthy of feeling better.

You also know, because I promise you it's true, that none of those things are more true than the fact that you deserve to feel better, and the people you love deserve to have the best-feeling version of you.

So the difference between those times and this time is that you know better, you know you're allowed to do better, and with the tools I'm giving you, you know *how* to do better.

> **Whether you flounder or flourish**
> **is always in your hands –**
> **you are the single biggest influence in your life.**
> **Oprah Winfrey –** *What I Know For Sure* [18]

Bill

Bill started a gratitude practice after his AA sponsor suggested it. He found immediate benefits for his mood, and his attitude towards his coworkers and boss, who he formerly considered "lame." He admitted he had gotten into such a bad habit of complaining to anyone who would listen, that he likely didn't know if anything was positive or not about his job or life. He was consistent with his new practice for a couple of months and clearly enjoyed the benefits, until he fell off the wagon. I asked him what happened and he said, "Who knows, I just don't feel like doing it anymore."

More questions revealed that Bill didn't feel comfortable feeling *that good*. He was enjoying a lot of positive results in his mood and outlook on life and had reached a new level of relief and joy. When I asked him again *why* he had stopped his gratitude practice, he said, "who am I to deserve this much happiness?" Bill had watched his father struggle all his life, get fired repeatedly, and eventually drink and smoke himself to death. Bill admitted he felt guilty (his *why not*) that he had found a path to sobriety before it was too late, and that he was feeling almost too optimistic about himself and his job, even hopeful about a possible promotion since his attitude had improved. I taught him EFT to release his guilt about doing better than his father, and helped him expand his comfort zone so he could "tolerate" more happiness and good fortune, and in time, reconnect to his gratitude practice.

Through Tapping, he also made the connection between his guilt and his sabotaging behavior – a form of punishment – whenever one of his friends from AA relapsed. He'd quit his gratitude practice and say he didn't deserve this much happiness when his friends were "sliding down the relapse hill." Using Tapping on a regular basis, Bill steadily increased his capacity for satisfaction at work and in life, for fulfillment in his relationships, and found a deeper connection to his community. He learned to have deep compassion for his friends who relapsed, and a more loving detachment from his father's "sad ending." He took responsibility for his own actions and his own happiness, and continued to use Tapping to treat the blocks to his joy. When he emptied his container of the negative memories, guilt, resentment, and fear, he was able to pick up his gratitude practice on a daily basis, and said he felt happier about his life than he had ever remembered.

CHAPTER 3

The Payoff

In Part 3, I will lead you through multiple EFT Tapping Sequences to help you release all three of your blocks: an emotional container that's been too full for too long; emotions and beliefs that show up as low self-esteem; and self-sabotaging behavior. But before I guide you to release them, we need to examine the real reasons for the third and final block: why you allow yourself to get in your own way.

*So what, exactly, are you trying to
protect yourself from – being visible?
Being successful? Being criticized?*

As I've said, we use self-sabotage for the purpose of emotional protection and safety. Getting to the right answers requires a deeper dive into the behavior, and more importantly, into the emotional conflicts and limiting beliefs that are driving the behavior.

In order to prepare you for using Tapping most effectively on self-sabotaging behaviors in the next section, we need to get to the underlying emotions and beliefs that are driving this behavior. When you get specific about the emotions and limiting beliefs that drive your compulsion to get in your own way, you'll be well on your way to solving and healing these cycles.

*Are you ready to take this deeper dive
into self-sabotage, get to the specific "why"
below the protection, and understand the bottom line?*

While self-sabotage is one of the primary blocks that kept me and keeps you from reaching for more emotionally expansive and helpful tools such as practicing gratitude, getting to the bottom of *why you sabotage yourself* will make the difference between a powerful and successful EFT practice and one that only scratches the surface.

Why do you stay stuck? Remember, there is a positive payoff from being stuck, blocking your success, and keeping a lid on your happiness, or you wouldn't do it. The positive intent is to protect you and keep you safe. Finding out what you need to shield yourself from will then prepare you for the EFT Sequences in the next section of the book.

Fears and limiting beliefs fuel your self-sabotaging behaviors – behaviors that keep you procrastinating, playing small, limiting your potential, and reining in your success.

These undermining behaviors obviously keep you going around in circles without getting anywhere, but most people just focus on hating themselves for having them.

**The payoff is substantial
or you wouldn't need to get in your own way.**

My container was way too full, my self-esteem was in the basement, and my self-destructive behavior was driving the external results in my life. It took incredible persistence to gain enough traction to be able to make substantial and fulfilling changes. What helped me dramatically was identifying what fears and beliefs drove this behavior – why I needed to stay safe from standing out.

If identifying your basic blocks and their costs has been enough to inspire you to change, you can start using the super tool of EFT in the next section to clear the path to practicing gratitude. However, many people, in spite of their enthusiasm for change, are unknowingly standing in their own way because there is a "payoff" to staying stuck or playing small.

If you're clear about what your blocks are and yet you still find yourself getting in your own way, you need to get to the bottom of the motivation that keeps you from welcoming and savoring the opportunity for more contentment and peace in your life. You may not have been aware that as much as you feel frustrated with getting in your own way, *there are good reasons for protecting yourself from moving forward.*

Below we'll examine the real reasons for this behavior by revisiting the primary questions I ask my clients when they feel stuck and can't seem to move forward.

1. What is the *upside* of staying stuck?
2. What is the *downside* of reaching your goals?

Basically, we're talking about your "setpoint" for happiness, health, and peace of mind. As an example of a setpoint, my biggest setpoint challenge for years was my weight. After a successful diet, I would bounce back up to my starting weight so fast my head would spin. I had a biological and emotional setpoint that made me feel more emotionally comfortable, so I easily and predictably returned to my comfort zone. *I wasn't ready to let go of the weight and create a new setpoint until I had identified and cleared what the upside of the extra weight and overeating behavior was for me – avoiding my feelings.* It wasn't until I discovered Tapping and worked on the deeper layers of grief and anxiety that I started to consistently lower my weight setpoint.

Most people don't realize that we also have setpoints for happiness, health, and peace of mind. This is where self-sabotage is running in the background, encouraging you to end a relationship, hand in inferior work, or be late to an important meeting.

Some people refuse to admit there's an upside to staying stuck. They have a list of excuses or reasons from outside of themselves – it's the economy, their boss, their spouse, or the professional climate in their field. But there are always opportunities and new paths you can take to excel at work, or options to exit an unhealthy job situation or relationship in a timely manner **- unless our feelings and beliefs keep us wed to staying stuck.**

Some people will claim there is absolutely no possible *downside* to feeling better or reaching their goals. Again, they often have a laundry list of excuses and reasons they can't possibly feel better. They remain passive, don't take control of what they can change, and claim they're a victim of circumstance.

This is my main theme in **The Yes Code**: keeping safe is the most important job our brains have been assigned. So, if feeling small, being less visible, or staying pessimistic makes you feel safe by protecting you from certain consequences, you will maintain that attitude and clip your level of success. Until you identify why you feel the need to keep yourself safe from being more visible, excelling, or feeling more joy or success, you can't treat the problem, and you will stay the same.

> *The real intent of self-sabotaging behaviors*
> *is to protect yourself from being exposed*
> *to some consequence you fear.*

Your emotional conflicts and limiting beliefs run the show: fear of success, fear of failure, fear of being visible, shining is unsafe, struggle is necessary, I need to play small. These fuel procrastination, perfectionism, people pleasing, addictions, and other forms of getting in your own way, *for the purpose of keeping yourself emotionally safe.*

Emotional Conflicts

Your blocks are all related. Unresolved emotional conflicts and traumatic memories from your childhood definitely fill your container, but they can also show up as low self-esteem in your relationships. Unresolved emotional blocks may also show up as addictions, fear of success or failure, and other self-defeating behaviors in adulthood. Your fears take up a lot of space in your container, but not only do they need to be cleared to make space in your container for more joy, they need to be cleared because they will show up in all aspects of your life.

For Example:

If you're scared of unpacking your childhood emotions – your grief, guilt, resentment, or betrayal – you may sabotage yourself as an adult by using substances or being engaged in busywork to protect yourself from having to feel your deep pain. You will feel safer, but will ultimately undermine your success.

If you're afraid to make a mistake because one of your caregivers was particularly harsh when you made a mistake as a child, you may develop the need for perfectionism in adulthood.

If you're afraid to shine because standing out as a child resulted in punishment or ridicule, you might sabotage yourself by steering yourself away from personal and professional opportunities in order to stay hidden under the radar.

If you were routinely judged and criticized as a child, you might sabotage yourself with procrastination, and find reasons to avoid writing your book, starting your new venture, or launching your YouTube channel.

__Holding back will protect you__
__from the exposure and potential criticism you fear.__

Limiting Beliefs

Your limiting beliefs come from the lessons you learned as a child. If your container is too full of painful childhood experiences that taught you how you "should" behave in order to stay safe, you're going to cling to these old beliefs as protection, even though you're an adult now and have control over many of your experiences.

If your family or teachers convinced you that you weren't smart enough to be successful, you will turn this belief into a self-fulfilling prophecy, sabotaging every chance at professional advancement that is offered to you. Then you will blame outside circumstances in order to avoid examining and changing your long-held beliefs.

If someone convinced you that you don't deserve what you want, you will sabotage your success by insisting there is negativity in every new situation, and be suspicious of positive opportunities offered to you in your personal and professional life.

If shining or standing out as a child ended in punishment or being the object of someone's jealousy, you will find creative ways to make excuses to keep a lid on your success because you're convinced being visible is unsafe.

Remember, the intent of self-sabotaging behavior is to keep you emotionally protected from something you fear. If you want to avoid the consequences of being successful, you'll procrastinate and waste time keeping busy but not really getting anything done. You'll miss deadlines, keep your goals out of reach, and blame your busy life for the interruptions and failures.

If you're afraid of someone's disapproval, you'll become a people-pleaser as a way to stay safe. People-pleasing will block you from setting appropriate boundaries and from confronting emotional conflicts in your relationships. Your relationships might appear to be conflict-free, but you'll feel unhappy and dissatisfied as a result.

Addictions are another way to sabotage yourself. If you don't lay off the sugar, alcohol, or cigarettes, you won't be as clear emotionally or intellectually, and will have more difficulty pursuing your goals. You may even get in trouble at work or at home because of your substance abuse. You'll blame stress, your family, your uncooperative boss, or your environment, but you'll keep cycling through addictions to keep you from feeling the emotions you need to address.

The behaviors (procrastination or perfectionism, addictions or neglecting your self-care) may look like the problem – but they are simply the result of the emotional conflicts and limiting beliefs you learned as a child. If you feel unsafe being successful, or believe standing out is dangerous, then hiding will serve a positive purpose. This cycle will keep you feeling safer from being exposed, but it will also keep you from reaching your goals and engaging with gratitude to allow yourself to be happier and healthier.

Janice

Janice made an appointment with me because she was shocked when she saw the number on the scale top her highest weight ever. She wondered how this slow creep up the scale had escaped her notice. When I asked her what had changed in her life, she mentioned her recent divorce battle and the frustration and helplessness leading up to it. She revealed that her husband had insinuated that their marriage was a casualty of her professional ambition. Ever since his comment during divorce proceedings she had been overeating and under-exercising. She was also showing signs of sloppiness at her job. Janice was using food to anesthetize her pain, grief, and the fear that her success ruined her marriage. The result was the inevitable extra weight.

When she became aware of the underlying reason for overeating, and acknowledged the purpose and positive intent of it, she started to accurately assess where she was, where she wanted to go, and most importantly, what she was going to do about it. She was able to use EFT effectively for her shame about her failed marriage, her intense late night cravings, and her tardiness at work that was putting a lid on her success.

As she started to acknowledge her painful feelings, take better care of herself, and improve her self-esteem, she was able to start a gratitude practice about her body and her life. While she initially felt very uncomfortable focusing on herself, she continued with the practice, made it a sacred part of her day, and combined Tapping with a mindful eating practice to lose and keep off the extra weight. Before, she secretly felt that she needed the safety and protection of using food and hating her body to keep her from feeling her emotional pain. It worked until the cost outweighed the benefit. Janice blossomed after committing to her gratitude practice – not only did she lose the weight she had gained, but she was more joyful, had more energy, and found herself much more compassionate with her friends, colleagues, and herself.

The Upside of Staying Stuck

Asking what the upside is to using gratitude as a daily practice isn't actually the right question, since we already know the answer: the benefits are incredible. The more revealing question is:

What is the upside of staying stuck?

That's the question that will identify the possible "payoff" of staying where you are: emotionally, physically, or in your relationships.

Why haven't you made any significant changes in your behaviors after months or years of unhappiness, complaints, and stories of who didn't do what when? It may be annoying to have to examine this, but it's the right thing to ask if you want to feel and be happier and more satisfied in your life.

Pamela

Pamela came to me to try and get sober. She said her entire life felt stuck, and she was finally able to admit that her drinking – not the people around her – was the problem. I asked her the upside of staying stuck for so long, and while she hated to admit it, she said it gave her an excuse to not have to face the "damage" she had done in her life while drinking. Staying stuck protected her from facing the emotional pain she felt about the hurt she had caused her parents, her siblings, and her boyfriend. She was stuck blaming other people, because she couldn't face the pain of her addiction. There was no way to make room for a gratitude practice when she was so full of pain.

She said that sure, she was grateful to be alive, but the rest of her life was a total mess. Once she admitted that there were emotions she didn't want to face, and that staying stuck kept her from feeling these painful emotions, she used Tapping for her shame, guilt, and fear of facing the damage she had caused. Tapping helped her stay present and calm, and she could own her "bizarre and scary" drunken behavior from her past. She could then turn her focus to what would be good about getting sober, and she was able to stick with counseling, AA, regular Tapping, her gratitude practice, and a joyful sober life.

If you're someone who might be using *being stuck* as a way to avoid feeling emotional pain, answer these foundational questions below about the ***upside of staying stuck:***

1. What is the upside of staying stuck?

_____
_____
_____

Some of the answers I have heard from my clients include:
- They won't expect anything from me.
- I can keep blaming forces outside of myself.
- I don't have to focus on painful feelings from my past.

2. How does staying stuck protect you?

_____
_____
_____

Some of the answers I have heard from my clients are:
- Staying stuck protects me from my own expectations.
- Staying stuck allows me to be attached to my struggle.
- Staying stuck helps me avoid painful emotions from childhood.

3. Is there any "payoff" to staying stuck and playing small in your personal life?

_____
_____
_____

Some of the answers I have heard from my clients are:
- I get to stay under the radar.
- No one will bother me about what I'm doing "next."
- I don't have to take responsibility for my own choices.

4. Is there any "payoff" to staying stuck and hiding in your professional life?

_____

_____

_____

Some of the answers I have heard from my clients include:
- Getting unstuck would come with more responsibilities.
- I can keep my head down and just get by.
- I don't have to be judged all the time.

5. What responsibilities and expectations do you avoid by staying the same?

_____

_____

_____

Some of the answers I have heard from my clients include:
- I get to avoid any new responsibilities.
- I don't have to unpack old trauma and grief.
- I get to stay comfortable instead of taking risks.

6. How does playing small benefit or "serve" you?

_____

_____

_____

Some of the answers I have heard from my clients include:
- Playing small and staying under the radar seem safer.
- Shining and being noticed would probably get me in trouble.
- I don't have to be afraid of failing at something new.
- I can avoid the usual expectations from my family.

7. Name at least 3 positive benefits of staying stuck (getting in your own way):

_____

_____

_____

Some of the answers I have heard from my clients include:
- I don't have to change.
- I don't have to examine my painful emotions.
- I won't be challenged.

Now that you have been alerted to a wide variety of feelings and beliefs that you might be using to stay safe, you can use the answers to these questions in the next section of the book where I teach you how to use Tapping on your emotions and beliefs.

The Downside of Reaching Your Goals

Asking what the downside is of being stuck is obvious too – it's frustrating, exhausting, and challenging. People claim it makes them unhappy and dissatisfied.

The more revealing question is:

> *What is the downside of reaching your goals,*
> *feeling happier, or getting what you want?*

When you answer this question, you will be identifying why you keep getting in your own way, and why you have yet to use a daily gratitude practice.

If you are frustrated with your situation yet haven't made significant changes, there must be a downside to feeling happier, more satisfied, or generally more content. If there wasn't a downside, you would be doing everything humanly possible to feel better, reach your goals, or take advantage of opportunities in your life. Maybe your setpoint is to have an "average" life, or to feel happy only some of the time. Maybe you don't feel you deserve much more than you have, or can only tolerate so much happiness.

*If your happiness and contentment are limited,
it only means your capacity is limited by emotional conflicts,
limiting beliefs, or self-sabotaging behavior.*

If you often witness yourself getting in your own way, it is evidence that you have unconsciously claimed a downside to being happier or reaching your goals. It doesn't matter whether you procrastinate, try to please others, avoid important conversations, or get distracted. The result is the same. You are keeping yourself from moving forward. To change directions, you need to ask the right questions and be honest about the answers.

*What is the downside of actually
reaching your goals and improving your life?*

John

John was bright and talented, dedicated to his family, and admittedly a little obsessed with being in good physical shape. He contacted me because he couldn't launch his website to attract clients for his new business coaching practice. He had left a corporate job at 40-something, and was excited to start doing performance coaching for executives. When I asked him what was stopping him from completing his website, he genuinely looked puzzled. "I can't figure it out. It's what I want!"

He told me he had started out eager, enthusiastic, and hopeful about his new profession, but when the opportunity came to put the finishing touches on his bio or launch the site, he always found himself running to the gym to lift weights. When I asked him if there was a possible downside to launching his website, he admitted that he was worried that some of his colleagues from his corporate job would think he was taking the easy road, instead of "toughing it out" in the corporate world. He was worried they would find his new job too "cushy."

When I asked if he thought this was what was blocking his forward momentum, he said he could tell it was by the queasy feeling he had in his stomach when talking about it. Once he identified this "downside" to launching his website, he was able to use EFT to release the fears and beliefs that were keeping him stuck, and was able to move forward and start attracting clients. Once his behavior was unpacked, he was able to add a gratitude practice to his self-care routine and enjoy the benefits of his new confidence almost immediately.

Answer the foundational questions below about the *downside* of being happier, healthier, and more successful:

1. What is the downside of being happier in your life?

_____

_____

_____

Some of the answers I have heard from my clients include:
- They'll expect more of me.
- I'll have to maintain it.
- It doesn't feel normal to be that happy.
- It's risky to be happier and get my hopes up.

2. How does avoiding success protect you?

_____

_____

_____

Some of the answers I have heard from my clients include:
- No one will notice me and be jealous.
- I don't have to have those uncomfortable conversations.
- I don't have to risk being visible.

3. What is the downside of standing out more in your personal life?

_____

_____

_____

Some of the answers I have heard from my clients include:
- My friends will be jealous.
- My colleagues will resent my happiness.
- I may become a target of their envy.

4. What is the downside of being more visible in your professional life?

_____

_____

_____

Some of the answers I have heard from my clients include:
- My colleagues will suspect my motives.
- I'll be teased for being the teacher's pet.
- It will take too much effort to "play the part."

5. If you were more successful, what responsibilities/expectations would you dread?

_____

_____

_____

Some of the answers I have heard from my clients include:
- Showing up more often.
- Making sure my work is perfect.
- They'll expect me to be a flawless employee.

6. Name at least 3 negative consequences of being more successful:

_____

_____

_____

Some of the answers I have heard from my clients include:
- I would have to keep up my new level of success.
- My mistakes would be more visible.
- I'll never be left alone.

7. How does being successful/more visible threaten or scare you?

_____

_____

_____

Some of the answers I have heard from my clients include:
- I'll always be in the spotlight.
- I'll have to be on guard all the time.
- I'll be open to attack from others who are jealous.
- People who stand out always get in trouble.

Now that you have identified the upside of staying stuck, and the downside of reaching your goals, you can address the real reasons you're blocking your happiness and satisfaction. Hopefully, this will give you more clues as to why you have been neglecting sticking to a gratitude practice in spite of the spectacular benefits.

Let's move on the next section where I will give a detailed overview of my favorite emotional technology – the tool of EFT – that will support you to empty your container of your painful past, improve your self-esteem by releasing the bad habits of devaluing yourself, and release the reasons for your chronic self-sabotaging behaviors.

The super-powerful tool of Tapping will clear the path so you can feel inspired to take advantage of the superpower of gratitude.

I will describe the origins of EFT Tapping, offer specific directions on how to use it most efficiently, and show you how to apply it to these main areas that keep you from taking better care of yourself. Then you can start and stick to a gratitude practice and enjoy its many benefits.

PART THREE
THE SOLUTION

CHAPTER 4
All About EFT Tapping

Now for the tool that changed my life and has changed the lives of thousands of people worldwide since it was created in the 1980's – the tool of Emotional Freedom Techniques (EFT) or what many people simply refer to now as "Tapping".

I have been a psychotherapist for 33 years, applying EFT on myself and my clients for 25 of those years. In my personal and professional experience, no other tool or "emotional technology" has ever come close to matching EFT's results for countless challenges, from stress relief to migraines, and from phobias to abundance issues. EFT is an exceptionally powerful tool, which, when used correctly, can help you take advantage of the superpower of gratitude I'm inviting you to incorporate into your life.

In this book, we're focusing on emptying your emotional container so you have room for more happiness, success, joy, and satisfaction; healing your low self-esteem; and eliminating the reasons you use self-sabotaging behaviors to stay safe. Below are some challenges that might be blocking you from sticking with self-care habits, such as a steady gratitude practice, that could make you feel much better – emotionally, physically, and even spiritually.

- Fear of success
- Fear of failure
- Fear of being visible
- Upsetting childhood events
- Generalized anxiety

- Guilt about your past
- Daily stress and conflicts
- Relationship conflicts
- Limiting beliefs about happiness
- Worthiness issues
- Low self-esteem
- Cravings
- Resentment

This one simple technique – EFT – can be used for all the fears, beliefs, past events, and memories that are blocking you from really feeling and being at your best. Whether you are afraid of being hurt again, or you are convinced you don't have what it takes, whether you were abandoned by loved ones, or feel guilty saying no, EFT will target your automatic emotional reactions and release the stress response in your brain that surfaces when you tune in to one of these feelings, beliefs, or memories.

The original method of tapping on acupuncture points was called Thought Field Therapy, and was created by a psychologist in California, Dr. Roger Callahan. Dr. Callahan found that by connecting to a client's acupuncture points through tapping with your fingertips, the brain would quiet down the fight or flight response that was triggered when focusing on a distressing topic. The brain would get rewired, and the usual anxiety response would decrease dramatically or disappear altogether.

Then Gary Craig, a Stanford-trained engineer and personal performance coach in California, simplified the complex "algorithms" of Dr. Callahan's original tapping prescriptions, and named his version of the tapping procedure "Emotional Freedom Techniques," or EFT. Most Tapping practitioners have been using this simplified version of Tapping since the 1990s.

What Is EFT or Tapping?

So, what exactly is this technique? EFT is essentially a stress management tool. It includes defined steps and a basic algorithm, originally called a recipe, where the clinician or the client uses their fingertips to tap on specific points on the face and body that correspond with traditional acupuncture points (acupoints) while repeating statements about the identified problem or distress. The location of the designated acupuncture points can be seen in the chart located later in this chapter.

In EFT, a simple, unified algorithm is used no matter what you are hoping to change or heal. If you want to change a feeling or belief, you're going to need to "call it up" in your mind first before tapping on these acupoints to relieve it. Just like editing a Word document, you'll need to open the file in order to make changes.

EFT includes identifying a problem, measuring the distress you feel connected to while tuning in to this problem, and then tapping on the acupuncture points (acupoints) to relieve the distress. Tuning in to the problem activates your stress response in relation to the problem you have identified. This means the feelings and beliefs are now "available" to be "edited" by using Tapping on the acupoints.

Tuning in to your distress activates the amygdala in your brain – the part of your brain we refer to as your "stress center" or your "smoke alarm." If the amygdala senses danger of any kind, it starts the alarm process and triggers your fight, flight, or freeze response. It can completely hijack your thoughts and focus when any stimulus *outside of you* reminds you of a past danger that has been recorded *inside of you.* Tapping with your fingertips on the acupoints calms the physiological response in your body that is triggered by recalling a painful memory in the past (maybe a memory associated with being visible or making a mistake), or by thinking of something worrisome in the future (maybe anticipating saying no to a colleague or family member). Tapping sends calming signals to the amygdala, and rewires the responses you have traditionally experienced from your personal triggers. EFT also lowers cortisol, the primary stress hormone, and releases endorphins, the feel good chemicals. All these effects take the emotional charge out of the topic you have chosen to release.

After decades of anecdotal success stories, some very dedicated clinicians and researchers have been tirelessly collecting data and completing studies that proved this method's effectiveness for fears, cravings, pain, and PTSD. Based on before and after responses, blood tests, saliva samples, and stress markers such as cortisol, the body of research studies has grown considerably. This research has changed the field, and allowed Clinical EFT and Tapping to become more widespread and accepted as a viable tool for clinicians and lay people for stress relief, anxiety, PTSD, pain, weight loss and more.[19][20][21][22]

Why and How It Works

The simple explanation for how EFT works is that combining Tapping on the acupoints with focusing on the emotional distress the person is feeling calms down the stress response – your fight or flight reaction – in your brain. Tapping on acupoints releases the emotional charge you normally experience when recalling a distressing event or thinking about a challenge in your future. For example, if you were previously afraid of contributing your ideas at a work meeting, after doing a few rounds of Tapping, the fear usually diminishes rapidly and permanently. The rewiring in the brain happens quite quickly with skillfully applied Tapping Rounds. Practitioners refer to what occurs during this process of calming down our distress in a variety of ways – rewiring, reprogramming, reintegrating, resolving, or refocusing. I call it rewiring the brain.

> *Stimulating acupuncture points (acupoints) by tapping on them while activating pertinent thoughts and feelings puts you at the keyboard as you reprogram the neural pathways that impact the quality of your life.*
>
> David Feinstein and Donna Eden, *Tapping*[23]

That's how simple an EFT Tapping session is: recall something stressful, tap on acupoints, and release the charge associated with the stressor. We are literally reprogramming the brain and rewiring your nervous system.

After many years of debate about how much of the success was attributable to the placebo effect, whether the clinician's personality mattered, and how ready the client was for healing, it has been shown through multiple research studies including fMRI imaging, that using Tapping on the acupoints is the "curative agent" in the treatment, as described in the books below. For those of you interested in a deeper dive into the mechanism of how EFT works and the research behind this technique, I highly recommend two must-read books in this field: Dr. Peta Stapleton's book, *The Science Behind Tapping*[24] and Dr. David Feinstein and Donna Eden's book, *Tapping*.[25]

If at any time during this process you feel overwhelmed with the emotions associated with your memories, please consult your health care provider for additional support.

How to Use Tapping Effectively

Once you learn the exact steps of EFT, the process is quite simple. When you follow the steps, you'll get results.

1. Choose your target.
2. Measure your fear or distress on the 0-10 point scale (10 is the highest level of stress or discomfort and 0 represents no stress or feeling neutral about the target).
3. Create a setup statement.
4. Tap on the acupoints while repeating the target you have chosen.
5. Re-test on the 0-10 point scale.
6. Repeat Tapping Rounds.

Choose Your Target

To conduct an effective round of Tapping, you'll need to choose a clear and specific **target**, or one of your blocks. Effective targets can be (1) an emotion, (2) a limiting belief, (3) a physical symptom, or (4) the memory of a past event. Here are some examples of each of these categories of targets.

Emotions

- I have a fear of being visible.
- I'm afraid of making a mistake.
- I'm afraid of being criticized.
- I have this fear of their jealousy.
- I'm afraid to face my past emotions.
- I'm afraid to fail if I try.
- I have this fear of being rejected.
- I'm afraid of feeling deep grief.
- I still feel hurt about the betrayal.
- I feel hurt about what he/she said to me.
- I feel resentful about what they said and did.
- I feel guilty when I say no.
- I feel guilty about my success.
- I feel guilty about letting them down.

Some examples of clear emotional targets from my life that I worked on with EFT included grief, fear of the other shoe dropping, fear of success, and guilt about my success.

Beliefs

- I'm convinced success isn't safe.
- Being visible is dangerous.
- I need to struggle like everyone else.
- I don't have what it takes to succeed.
- I'm too old to change.

- I'm convinced they'll attack me if I'm successful.
- All relationships are trouble.
- Standing out will get me noticed too much.
- It's safe to stay under the radar.
- Playing small is safer.
- I'm not worth time and attention.

Some of the beliefs I worked on from my story included the belief that I didn't deserve to be happier, the belief that standing out was unsafe, and the belief that being visible would get me in trouble.

Symptoms

- I have a throbbing headache.
- I have this pain in my knee.
- I have this intense pain in my lower back.
- I have this tension in my neck.
- I have intense sugar cravings.
- My bloated stomach bothers me.
- I suffer from numbness in my feet.

Symptoms I have worked on to improve my life included sugar cravings, headaches, fatigue, and weakness as a result of low blood sugar.

Memory of a Past Event

- The time my teacher humiliated me in front of the class.
- The time my friend said I didn't deserve what I had.
- The time I felt hurt by their criticism.
- The time they mocked me for being visible.
- The time my grandmother said I couldn't be successful.
- The time my father yelled at me in front of my friends.

My primary targets of past events I needed to work on from my life included getting an upsetting medical diagnosis, the shock of a car accident, memories of my mother's relapses, memories of the phone calls informing me someone had died, and memories of being hurt because someone was jealous of my success.

Measure Your Stress Level

You've chosen your target – a feeling, belief, symptom, or memory – and now you need to measure how high your stress feels to you on a particular topic when you tune in to it on the 0-10 point scale. On this scale, 10 represents the highest level of distress, and 0 represents a feeling of neutrality about the target.

The point of using the 0-10 point intensity scale, (originally called the "SUDS" level – subjective units of distress) is to accurately measure the baseline level of fear or stress that you feel about the original target so you can measure again after you have completed the treatment to make sure the Tapping is working. If your number isn't decreasing, it's a good indication that you need to adjust your target or the words you are using.

For instance, if you are afraid to stand out because you worry that someone will attack you, you would measure how afraid you feel on the 0-10 point scale when you think of standing out now, and then re-measure your fear after each round of Tapping.

Create Your Setup Statement

The **setup statement** is a clear description of the fear, belief, symptom, or memory, followed by a phrase of acceptance. Let's say you've chosen your target as the fear of making a mistake. You've brought this fear to mind and measured your distress on the 0-10 point scale, and it measures as a 7. In this example, the setup statement would sound like this: *"Even though I'm afraid of making a mistake, I deeply and completely love and accept myself anyway."* We will repeat this setup statement while we tap on the first acupoint, the side of the hand (or karate chop point). But first, let's look at some classic setup statements.

These setup statements include a description of the problem (the target) and a phrase of acceptance. In the examples below, the targets are underlined. The original acceptance phrase used by clinicians worldwide was *I deeply and completely love and accept myself.* Over the years, clinicians became more flexible with this phrase of acceptance in order to meet their clients' comfort levels. As a result, new practitioners and lay people use a wide variety of acceptance phrases at the end of their setup statements. The point is to pair the description of the problem with a statement of compassion and acceptance. Below I have included a variety of acceptance phrases. When in doubt, you can always default to the original phrase of acceptance at the end of every setup statement: *I deeply and completely love and accept myself.*

Even though <u>I feel afraid of standing out too much</u>, I deeply and completely love and accept myself.

Even though <u>I've always been afraid of shining</u>, I understand why and accept myself anyway.

Even though <u>I feel afraid of failing</u>, I accept who I am and how I feel about this possibility.

Even though <u>I feel afraid of feeling my deep grief</u>, I accept who I am and how I feel about this topic.

Even though <u>I have intense cravings for sugar</u>, I deeply and completely accept myself and my reaction.

Even though <u>I feel upset when I remember what happened back then</u>, I accept who I am and how I feel about it.

Even though <u>I feel guilty when I consider saying no</u>, I choose to feel calm and peaceful anyway.

Even though <u>I feel resentful when I think of how hard I'm working</u>, I accept who I am and where I learned this.

Even though <u>I feel afraid of making a mistake</u>, I accept my whole body and appreciate how strong it is.

Even though <u>they convinced me that I'll never be good enough</u>, I accept who I am and how I feel anyway.

Even though <u>I'm convinced that playing small is safer</u>, I accept who I am and where I learned this.

Even though <u>I'll never forget being humiliated in front of everyone</u>, I accept who I am and how I feel.

Tapping On Acupoints

To begin this process, we use two fingers to tap on the side of the hand while repeating the setup statement two or three times. Then we proceed to the additional Tapping points on the face and body, repeating the target phrase. Most people tap with two fingers of their primary hand. (I'm right-handed so I tap with the two fingers of my right hand.) You can tap on one side of the face and body; it's not necessary to tap on both sides. And you don't need to tap very hard – not as hard as knocking on a door, but about as hard as tapping someone on the shoulder. All you need to do is make physical contact with the acupoint located right below the skin.

The next step is to identify your target phrase, "I'm afraid to make a mistake," in this case, and tap on the series of acupoints listed below while repeating this phrase. Here is a list of the remaining points where you will tap and repeat the original target you chose. (See chart below).

Eyebrow

Side of Eye

Under Eye

Under Nose

Chin

Collarbone

Under Arm

Head

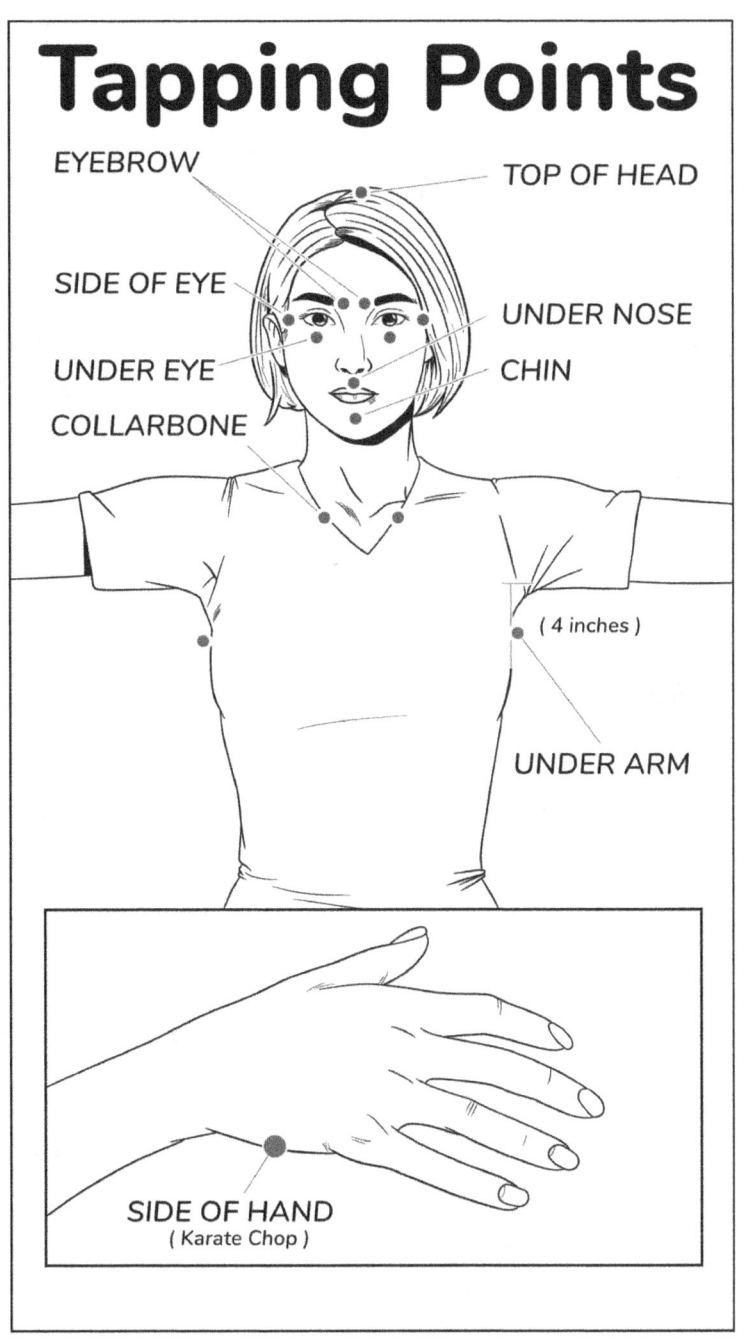

The order of the Tapping points works for simplicity, so if you change the order, it won't reduce the effectiveness of your Tapping Round. You may also change the wording (as long as you stay on the general topic) so that repeating "I'm afraid of making a mistake" several times doesn't feel too monotonous to you. Beginners can follow this protocol and repeat the exact same target phrase at each point and get excellent results.

Re-Test Distress

After completing the setup statement and one full round of Tapping on each of the remaining acupoints – this is called a Tapping Round or Tapping Sequence – you will tune in to your original target and measure the distress you feel again on the same 0-10 point scale. Usually, the initial feeling of fear or distress will have decreased at least a few points. If not, either reword the target, get more tuned in to the stressor you chose to work on, or keep repeating the original simple Tapping Round. Sometimes the target has moved – while you were first tuned in to feeling afraid of making a mistake, you now feel stressed about being exposed in front of your boss. You may adjust the words to describe your target accordingly.

I will be providing dozens of Tapping Scripts in Chapters 5-8 to address your fears, beliefs, symptoms, and memories of any past events that have limited your emotional container for joy and happiness.

Review

To review, a typical Tapping Round or Sequence includes the following steps:

1. **Choose your target** (an emotion, a belief, a symptom, or a memory of an event).
2. **Measure your fear or distress** on the 0-10 point scale (where 10 represents the highest amount of distress or discomfort and 0 represents feeling neutral about the topic).
3. **Create a setup statement** and repeat it out loud while tapping on the point on the side of your hand (karate chop point).

4. **Tap on the remaining acupoints** while repeating your **target phrase**.

5. Re-test your fear or distress on the 0-10 point scale.

6. Repeat Tapping Rounds until your number on the scale is low enough for you to move onto another topic.

Putting It All Together:

Choose your target: In the sample Tapping Round below, I will be using *I'm afraid to be visible* as the target.

Measure how high your stress feels to you on the 0-10 point scale.

Create your setup statement: Even though I'm afraid to be visible, I deeply and completely love and accept myself anyway.

Start tapping on the side of your hand while you repeat the setup statement: Even though I'm afraid to be visible, I deeply and completely love and accept myself anyway. Even though I'm afraid to be visible, I accept who I am and how I feel.

Tap on the series of remaining acupoints while saying the target phrase (or variations of the original target).

> **Eyebrow:** I'm afraid to be visible.
> **Side of Eye:** I'm afraid to shine and be visible.
> **Under Eye:** I feel stress about it in my body.
> **Under Nose:** I'm afraid to be visible.
> **Chin:** I don't want to stand out.
> **Collarbone:** If I shine, I might get into trouble.
> **Under Arm:** I don't want to be visible.
> **Head:** No wonder I hold myself back.

Re-test how high your fear about the target feels to you now on the 0-10 point scale. Continue Tapping on this target until your distress decreases enough that you feel comfortable moving on to another target.

Tapping Guidelines

I recommend to all my clients that they aim to use Tapping between 10-20 minutes a day, rain or shine. When you use Tapping on yourself to release old feelings of hurt, guilt, resentment and fear, the results will create momentum for you to take better care of yourself. As you clean out your emotional container, you'll be able to expand your capacity to embrace more joy, freedom, and happiness. As you release the events or memories that caused you to feel low self-esteem, you'll want to reach for better self-care habits. And as you identify and release the reasons you are using self-sabotaging behavior, you'll be inspired to take even better care of yourself and stick with other self-care practices, such as writing your daily gratitude lists, or gratitude journaling.

You may choose a fear or belief that you know has been holding you back from more joy in your life, or choose something stressful that happened during the day at work or at home. You could choose something that concerns you in the near future, or a memory of a past event. ***The point is to be specific when you're choosing your target, and dedicate time to this daily practice.***

If you are targeting a fear of standing out, and your intensity number starts at an 8 and then drops to a 4, you may feel ready to move onto another target. Some people insist on getting the fear down to a 0-1, but it's up to you. When you get your stress to a low enough number, you'll feel ready to choose another Tapping Target or complete your Tapping Rounds for the day. If there is still an emotional charge on the fear or belief you were Tapping on, it's an indication that you have more Tapping work to do. Keep using the 0-10 point measurement scale until you feel confident that the fear, belief, symptom, or memory has subsided.

If you are struggling with work or family stress, use those topics as your targets and put aside Tapping time every day.

If you're about to have a challenging meeting with your boss, I would use Tapping several times before the meeting, including the day before.

If you're going to visit your family, and you're afraid they're going to criticize you, I would use the Tapping for a couple of days before you go. In addition, you could find a quiet space or go into the bathroom and use a few minutes of Tapping to calm yourself down during your visit. Don't forget to measure your fear before and after the Tapping.

If you have struggled with high cravings for sugar or any substance, I always tell my clients, "Don't wait until you're on your way to Dunkin' Donuts" because trust me, you won't start Tapping. This is why I recommend having a daily Tapping practice instead of waiting until a crisis. When you feel urgent about something, your brain will be hijacked and you won't remember to reach for the Tapping process.

If particularly upsetting memories about traumatic events surface while you are Tapping, please consult a qualified healthcare practitioner for support.

Gratitude Tapping

After studying and using exercises around gratitude and appreciation, I created and added the simple practice of Gratitude Tapping and Thank You Tapping to my EFT work, and many practitioners have caught on to this variation.

The power of gratitude is that it sends a "Yes, thank you!" to the Universe.

Again, wait until you've decreased your distress about the topic you chose at least by a few points before moving on to Gratitude Tapping. Gratitude Tapping helped me stick to my gratitude practice because it felt relaxing, fun, and helped me end the Tapping Sequences with total joy. Gratitude Tapping Phrases while tapping on the acupoints are phrases like:

- I'm so grateful that we resolved the conflict.
- I appreciate what I've learned from this experience.
- I'm thankful for the relationship we had.

- Thank you, Universe (or use God, Higher Power, Infinite Intelligence), for sending me or bringing me the solution to this problem.
- Thank you for bringing me the solution to this problem.
- Thank you for so many supportive friends.
- Thank you for the resolution to this conflict.

In the next section of the book, I will be providing numerous Tapping exercises focused on clearing the three primary blocks to sticking with the superpower of gratitude:

1. Your container is too full.
2. You have low self-esteem.
3. You engage in self-sabotaging behavior.

These exercises will support you to release these blocks, feel more emotionally free and confident, and help you more easily stick with your daily gratitude practice.

Scan this QR code or visit your *Yes, Thank You* book portal at www.theyescode.com/thankyou to review EFT Videos and other supporting materials for this book.

CHAPTER 5
Your Container Is Full

An emotional container full of old garbage is one of the main problems for so many people: there's just not enough room to hold more joy and contentment. If this is one of your challenges, then Tapping is the solution to clear these emotional blocks. Tapping will help you clear out your emotional conflicts and past memories so you'll feel much lighter emotionally, and then you are more likely to take advantage of what self-care tools are available to you.

Like the dieter who relapses with sugar on a Tuesday, has a hard time getting back on the bike on Wednesday, and throws in the towel on Thursday, the negative cycle builds momentum and sometimes it's incredibly hard to pump the brakes. However, the cycle moves in the other direction as well. *Once you feel better, you do better things for yourself,* which makes you feel even better, and the momentum for looking for ways to feel joy and happiness improves. When you use Tapping to clear out your past feelings and memories from your emotional container, you will have space to fill with the benefits of a steady gratitude practice.

Your Container Is Too Full

Let's begin with our EFT Tapping to heal the blocks that are getting in the way of taking care of yourself. When you feel weighed down by emotional conflicts or memories from your past, these feelings and memories interfere with your drive to take care of yourself, which in turn blocks you from expanding your container for joy and happiness.

Below I will address numerous old feelings and memories that might be in your container, so you can start the process of making space for more joy, happiness, and contentment.

For each Tapping Target, I have provided two Tapping Sequences to address the specific emotion or negative memory, followed by a Gratitude Tapping Sequence to help you combine the truth about the problem with a focus towards expressing what you appreciate.

Tapping Target: Family Conflict

As I told you in the section called My Story, I was so preoccupied with chaos and pain in my family, I wasn't focused on taking care of myself. With this focus, I wasn't able to avail myself of self-care practices like a daily gratitude practice. Until I could change the balance of my focus to helping myself feel better, I couldn't focus on what I needed. I had to clean out the negative thoughts and the mental preoccupation before I could make more room for joy and contentment.

Often, we let a past family conflict interfere with our peace of mind in our current life. The memory might feel very alive now. Or even though it's been decades since it happened, the past conflict might feel as if it is very present. Try this Tapping Sequence below.

When you think of the distress you feel about a particular family conflict (in the past or present), measure how high your stress level is on the 0-10 point scale. Then start using Tapping:

Side of Hand: Even though I'm so upset about this family conflict, I deeply and completely love and accept myself anyway. Even though I feel upset about this family conflict, I accept who I am and how I feel.
Eyebrow: I'm so upset by what's happening (happened) in my family.
Side of Eye: I'm very upset about my family conflict.
Under Eye: I feel so much distress right now.
Under Nose: I can't focus on myself.
Chin: I want to help them.

Collarbone: I'm so preoccupied with my family.
Under Arm: I want to find a solution to the conflict.
Head: I feel so distracted by my family situation.

Take a deep breath, and check the stress you feel about this family situation on the 0-10 point scale again. Continue with your Tapping:

Side of Hand: Even though I'm still so worried about my family situation that I can't even concentrate, I accept who I am and how I feel. Even though I'm so preoccupied by my family distress, I accept how I feel and where my focus is.
Eyebrow: I'm still so worried about my family situation.
Side of Eye: I can't concentrate on anything else.
Under Eye: I'm still really worried about my family situation.
Under Nose: I'm still worried it won't turn out well.
Chin: I'm concerned and worried about the problem.
Collarbone: I still can't focus on myself.
Under Arm: I don't want to focus on myself.
Head: I'm so worried about my family.

Take a deep breath, and measure your stress and concern you still feel about the family situation on the 0-10 point scale. You may continue Tapping with the above sequences, change the wording to better suit your specific situation, or substitute another concern in the phrasing. When you feel ready, proceed to the Gratitude Tapping Sequence below.

Side of Hand: Even though I still feel concerned about my family situation, I deeply and completely love and accept myself anyway. Even though I'm still worried about my family situation, I choose to remember how grateful I am.
Eyebrow: I feel worried, but I still feel grateful.
Side of Eye: I appreciate my family.
Under Eye: Thank you for my entire family.
Under Nose: I appreciate that they're doing the best they can.
Chin: Thank you, Universe for so much to appreciate about my family.

Collarbone: I'm grateful for my family.
Under Arm: Thank you, Universe, for so many blessings.
Head: Thank you for all that I have to appreciate about my life.

Take a final deep breath, and measure your level of stress now on the 0-10 point scale about the first issue you chose as your focus. Continue using the Tapping Sequences above until you feel more balanced about the situation that is concerning you.

Disagreements

Having an argument with a loved one is very emotionally time-consuming. Even when you're not with that person, you're thinking about the argument, how it went, how it will go, will it ever get resolved, who's right and who's wrong, etc. Using Tapping can take the sting out of the argument, help you feel clearer, and know whether to salvage the relationship, or cut your losses and move on. People either agree to disagree, continue the fight for years, or they split their relationship altogether. I've seen every variation and outcome. Yes, some arguments are unresolvable, but before you make any decisions to end a relationship, I invite you to do some dedicated Tapping work.

Marla

Marla had been attending her therapy sessions weekly for at least 6 months before she revealed to me that she was having a "standoff" with her cousin, who she said was more like a sister to her. When I asked what the argument was about, she said it centered around her cousin criticizing Marla about how she was raising her children. Her cousin voiced the concern that Marla and her husband were too relaxed about certain boundaries and discipline with their children, including how they let them talk back to their parents. The cousin said, "we weren't raised that way" and blamed Marla's husband. Stuck in between her cousin and husband, Marla had pushed back with "you don't know anything about raising kids" and refused to listen to her cousin's point of view. To make it more complicated, Marla and her husband regularly relied on this cousin for babysitting, filling in when they both worked late. The kids adored her and didn't mind some of her stricter rules around bedtime and watching tv.

Marla already knew about Tapping, as I had taught her to use it when she and her husband fought, and when she had trouble setting boundaries with her boss. Part of why her cousin had to frequently pick up the kids after school was that Marla had difficulty saying no to her boss when he asked her for last minute favors at the end of the day. When I suggested Marla write a gratitude list about her cousin, she was furious. "She's being a real bitch right now, so, no thanks." Marla said she didn't want to give in, and that she had been working hard to stand up for herself and didn't want to cave on this point. I explained to Marla that I wasn't asking her to cave in, give in, or not stand up for herself. But that along with her Tapping on her anger, writing a gratitude list would calm her down so that she could start to see more of her cousin's perspective with neutrality, and ask for space to share her own views. She still wouldn't budge. We kept using Tapping on her anger and frustration, and her uncomfortable experience of feeling trapped between her husband and her favorite cousin.

One week she came into her appointment and said: "OK, I wrote your stupid gratitude list!" The outcome? She admitted she knew her cousin had important points about her boundaries with her kids, loosened some of the sting from being hurt, and was willing to talk to her cousin. She was able to have that conversation, express her feelings, state her gratitude about everything this cousin did for her, and still maintain her boundary that she wasn't interested in her opinions about how she and her husband were raising their kids. Did her gratitude list save the day? No, but it made her more neutral on the topic, able to see both sides, and she was able to thaw out the block of ice that had developed between the two of them, and resume their relationship without resentment. She became a fan of writing gratitude lists and encouraged her husband and kids to write them as well.

Tapping Target: Argument With a Loved One

Try this Tapping Sequence about an argument or disagreement with a loved one.

Measure how frustrated, annoyed, or angry you feel now towards the other person on the 0-10 point scale, even though the argument may have occurred years ago. Start your Tapping:

Side of Hand: Even though I feel frustrated and irritated that they wouldn't see my point of view, I deeply and completely love and accept myself anyway. Even though I felt so annoyed that he/she wouldn't see what they did, I accept who I am and how I feel about it.

Eyebrow: I'm so frustrated by this argument.
Side of Eye: They won't hear my side.
Under Eye: They don't get it.
Under Nose: I'm tired of fighting.
Chin: But I don't want to back down.
Collarbone: I need to stand up for myself.
Under Arm: I'm tired of the argument.
Head: The truth is I feel hurt and misunderstood.

Take a deep breath and measure how frustrated, hurt, or angry you feel now about the argument on the 0-10 point scale. Continue your Tapping:

Side of Hand: Even though I still feel frustrated by this fight I'm having/I had with _____, I deeply and completely love and accept myself anyway. Even though I'm still frustrated that they won't back down, I accept who I am and how I feel.

Eyebrow: I'm still mad about the whole thing.
Side of Eye: I'm still frustrated about how it started.
Under Eye: I'm still frustrated by this argument.
Under Nose: It's not getting better.
Chin: I'm still frustrated and hurt.
Collarbone: I don't see how it's going to be resolved.
Under Arm: I feel anxious about the separation I feel.

Head: I feel hurt and anxious about the argument.

Take another deep breath, and measure your feelings about the argument and that person now on the 0-10 point scale. If your level of frustration or hurt is still over a 6, I would recommend that you continue using Tapping on these feelings. You may change the wording to better suit your specific situation. When you feel ready, proceed to the Gratitude Tapping below.

Side of Hand: Even though I still feel angry and hurt about the argument, I feel grateful for this relationship and I'm open to hearing his/her side. Even though I still feel hurt about the words we exchanged, I accept who I am and how I feel.
Eyebrow: I'm grateful we had the fight.
Side of Eye: I'm grateful we aired our differences.
Under Eye: Thank you, Universe, for this great relationship.
Under Nose: Thank you for such a good resolution.
Chin: Thank you, Universe, for a solution to this fight.
Collarbone: I'm grateful I can see his/her point.
Under Arm: I'm grateful he/she is willing to see my point.
Head: Thank, you, Universe, for bringing me such a peaceful resolution.

Take a final deep breath, and measure your feelings now about the argument on the 0-10 point scale. You may tap on any aspect of the argument – how it started, why it started, the words that were expressed, your regret about what you said – until you feel ready to approach the other person with an open mind and heart.

Grief

Whether you're suffering from the loss of a job, a relationship, a pet or losing a loved one, grief can show up in many different ways. While there is the common format from Elisabeth Kubler-Ross's book about the 5 stages of grief,[26] there are no actual linear "stages" of grief, as anyone knows who has lived through a profound loss. When we've lost a loved one and are feeling the deep pain and sorrow, it can be very challenging to get enough sleep and regular meals, much less engage in self-care practices such as keeping a gratitude diary.

In hindsight, I wish I had been able to write a gratitude list when my mother died so suddenly, but I wasn't anchored in the practice enough for it to be a "go to" tool during those dark times. Moving through the pain of grief takes time – lots of time – and while your feelings will change, the grief process never really *ends*. If you open yourself up enough to love in your life, you'll end up grieving losses. Using Tapping helped me clear remaining bits of regret and guilt, release the pain of the sorrow, and helped me focus on appreciation instead of just pain.

Jackie

Jackie lost her mother after a long illness that included many ups and downs with the assisted living arrangements. Not only was she grieving, but she also described herself as "bone tired" and somewhat numb. She knew she should be full of sorrow, but the harrowing last few years had left her feeling so depleted she didn't actually feel sad. The Tapping helped thaw her out from feeling depleted and run down, and she was soon able to acknowledge that all her feelings connected to her mother's death were "appropriate" even if they didn't follow a particular path.

Restoring her emotional health and regular schedule needed to be a priority before she could really honor the enormous loss she felt. In addition, she felt relief. Her mother had suffered terribly, and Jackie felt resentful that her siblings hadn't helped enough with their mother's care. Jackie felt relieved not only that her mother was out of pain, but also that she didn't have to spend all her waking time checking to make sure the assisted living staff was taking care of her.

While her relief was understandable, she felt enormous guilt about her relief, and didn't share it with her siblings or friends for fear she would be criticized. In our sessions together, I was able to help Jackie normalize the wide range of emotions she was experiencing, and she learned to respect every part of the painful but necessary grieving process. She enjoyed the Tapping

Sequences on the different angles of her grief, and was quickly able to feel grateful for her relationship with her mother, and the freedom she had that enabled her to contribute to her care.

Tapping Target: Grief

Consider the current or past grief that has your attention right now. If you have suffered many losses, try to isolate one of them for this exercise. Measure the level of sorrow or loss you feel on the 0-10 point scale, and proceed:

Side of Hand: Even though I feel heartbroken about my loss, I accept who I am and how I feel. Even though I feel such deep sorrow about my loss, I deeply and completely love and accept myself anyway.

Eyebrow: I feel such profound grief right now.

Side of Eye: I feel sad all the time.

Under Eye: I feel this deep grief.

Under Nose: I can't focus on anything else.

Chin: I feel such deep grief.

Collarbone: It feels like I'm falling apart.

Under Arm: This deep grief.

Head: I can't focus on anything else.

Take a deep breath, and measure your grief now on the 0-10 point scale. Some people admit to feeling resistance to reducing their grief. They worry that if they don't feel as sad as they think they should, it means they didn't care that much about their loved one. If you find yourself feeling resistant to feeling better, consider this conflict and notice what surfaces in your Tapping Sequences. You may always devise new Tapping Sequences that match your experience. Continue with your Tapping:

Side of Hand: Even though I still feel like I'm drowning in my grief, I deeply and completely love and accept myself anyway. Even though my grief still feels overwhelming to me, I accept who I am and how I'm handling this loss.

Eyebrow: I feel such deep grief right now.

Side of Eye: I can't seem to focus on anything else.
Under Eye: I feel so sad about my loss.
Under Nose: I miss him/her so much.
Chin: The pain and grief are so intense.
Collarbone: I feel so much pain and sorrow.
Under Arm: I feel heartbroken and sad.
Head: I feel such deep grief.

Take a deep breath, and measure the level of pain and grief you feel now on the 0-10 point scale. Remember, it might feel uncomfortable to feel better, but it does not mean you didn't love the person. It just means you are processing the variety of emotions that surface during the grieving process and allowing yourself more balance. If you thought of more conflicts or challenges about the grieving process, you may formulate new target statements and use them at a later time.

Proceed to this final Gratitude Tapping Round.

Side of Hand: Even though I still feel the pain of loss, I appreciate all that we had together. Even though it's hard to remember the good times right now, I am grateful for the love and connection we felt.
Eyebrow: I'm grieving but I feel grateful for what we had.
Side of Eye: I appreciate so much about the relationship.
Under Eye: I appreciated him/her so much.
Under Nose: I loved who I was with her/him.
Chin: Thank you, Universe, for bringing her/him into my life.
Collarbone: I feel so grateful for our relationship.
Under Arm: Thank you, Universe, for bringing her/him into my life.
Head: Thank you, Universe, for so many blessings about this relationship.

Take a deep breath and measure your grief now on the 0-10 point scale.

You may use this series of Tapping Sequences for a specific loss, or for an overall or generalized feeling of grief and loss in your life. I invite you to end each round with Gratitude Tapping, using your own words.

Anger

Think about your past. Do you feel angry about your past? Anger at your parents, siblings, the situations you were in? For some people, anger feels strong and clarifying. It makes them feel justified and grounded. But at what point is the old anger hurting your peace of mind and health?

Tapping Target: Anger

Think of a situation you feel angry or helpless about, or a person you blame for something that happened in your past. Now measure how angry you feel on the 0-10 point scale, all these years later, at that person when you think of the event. Start the Tapping Sequence below:

Side of Hand: Even though I feel angry at this person because it was his/her fault, I accept who I am and how I feel about it. Even though I feel angry that they didn't protect me, I accept who I am and how I feel.

Eyebrow: I feel so angry about it.
Side of Eye: I hate what happened.
Under Eye: Why didn't they protect me?
Under Nose: I feel so angry about what happened.
Chin: I'm so mad they didn't take care of me.
Collarbone: I still feel angry about it.
Under Arm: I don't want to let it go.
Head: Then they'd win.

Take a deep breath, and measure how angry you feel at that same person now on the 0-10 point scale. If you feel some resistance to letting it go, that's ok, but you'll need to identify why you feel the need to hold onto it, what it's costing you, and whether you are willing to let it go or not.

Side of Hand: Even though I still feel angry about what happened in my childhood, I deeply and completely love and accept myself anyway. Even though I still feel angry at this person for what she/ he said and did, I accept my feelings and the situation.

Eyebrow: I still feel so angry about it.

Side of Eye: I'm afraid to let it go.
Under Eye: I still feel so angry at her/him.
Under Nose: I'm reluctant to let it go.
Chin: I never want to forgive them.
Collarbone: And that's my right.
Under Arm: But I'd like to release some of the anger.
Head: It's exhausting me and I'm tired of it.

Take a deep breath, and measure your anger about this exact situation or person again on the 0-10 point scale. When you feel ready, proceed to the Gratitude Tapping below. If it feels too uncomfortable to you, I recommend completing some more basic rounds on your levels of anger.

Side of Hand: Even though I still feel angry and unable to forgive, at least I accept my feelings and how I got here. Even though I still feel angry and unwilling to forgive, I deeply and completely love and accept myself anyway.
Eyebrow: I'm still angry, but I appreciate myself.
Side of Eye: I'm grateful for all that I've learned.
Under Eye: I feel grateful that I've matured so much.
Under Nose: I feel thankful that I'm not still in that situation.
Chin: I'm grateful that so much has changed.
Collarbone: Thank you, Universe, for bringing me a better perspective.
Under Arm: Thank you for showing me what I could appreciate.
Head: I'm grateful to be back in control of my life now.

Take a deep breath, and measure how angry you still feel now on the 0-10 point scale towards this person or about the situation. The feelings of anger and helplessness often go together, and in fact, sometimes feeling the strength of anger feels like an antidote to helplessness. If this feels true for you, you could substitute feeling angry with helplessness and start with this setup statement: "Even though I felt so helpless back then, I deeply and completely love and accept myself anyway."

Guilt

I've worked with clients in workshops about guilt over what they've said, done, didn't do, and how they feel about their actions. I often start by asking: "And how long have you felt this guilt?" Many have answered "for decades."

Tapping Target: Guilt

Do you have a strong feeling of guilt from your past? Guilt that you didn't say the right thing or do the right thing, or guilt that you did something you were told was "wrong"? Measure that feeling of guilt now on the 0-10 point scale and start Tapping:

Side of Hand: Even though I feel so guilty about what I said and did back then, I deeply and profoundly love and accept myself anyway. Even though I feel so guilty about what I said and did back then, I accept who I am now.

Eyebrow: I'm tortured by my guilt.
Side of Eye: I think about it all the time.
Under Eye: I feel so guilty about what I did and said.
Under Nose: I feel so guilty and think about it all the time.
Chin: I feel incredibly guilty about what I said and did back then.
Collarbone: I really beat myself up with the guilt.
Under Arm: I wish I had done it differently.
Head: I still feel a lot of guilt.

Take a deep breath and measure how guilty you feel now on the 0-10 point scale about what happened. Continue with the next round:

Side of Hand: Even though I still feel guilty for what happened back then, and I wish I had done it differently, I deeply and completely love and accept myself anyway. Even though I still feel guilty for what I said and did, and I wish I could take it back, I deeply and completely love and accept myself anyway.

Eyebrow: I wish I could take it back.
Side of Eye: I wish I hadn't said what I said.
Under Eye: I wish I hadn't done what I did.

Under Nose: I feel so guilty.
Chin: I feel so much guilt and regret.
Collarbone: I wish I could change what happened.
Under Arm: I still feel guilty no matter what.
Head: I wish I could change it.

Take another deep breath, and measure how guilty you feel now about what happened, on the 0-10 point scale. Once the intensity on this incident has been reduced, another incident may grab your attention. Stick to this original one until your guilt measures much lower on the 0-10 point scale, and then return to the Tapping Sequences with your new incident or memory in your mind. Proceed to the Gratitude Tapping.

Side of Hand: Even though I still feel guilty about what happened, I'm going to consider letting some of the guilt go now. Even though I still feel guilty for what I said and did back then, I choose to release some of it now.
Eyebrow: I still feel guilty, but I appreciate who I've become.
Side of Eye: I appreciate so much about my life.
Under Eye: I want to stop feeling guilty and appreciate who I am.
Under Nose: I choose to appreciate who I've become.
Chin: I'm so grateful for my life now.
Collarbone: Thank you, Universe, for all the lessons I learned.
Under Arm: I'm grateful for all the lessons I've learned.
Head: Thank you for so much to appreciate about my life.

Take a final deep breath, and measure your guilt now on the 0-10 point scale. If another incident surfaces for you, you may substitute the details in your next Tapping Rounds.

Fear

I lived in fear – fear of my parents' drinking, fear of a car accident, fear of being yelled at...the list was long. In my early adulthood, even though I was totally independent, the fear and memories about the frightening things that did happen were still lodged in my nervous system; they were just out of sight because I was no longer in the situation. My Tapping work changed my nervous system and my outlook on my life.

Tapping Target: Fear

Think of a particular fear you have now, or a memory of a fearful event from your past. If you can still get an emotional charge on it, that is an indication that it's still clogging your container. Measure how fearful you feel about the memory now, on the 0-10 point scale. Then start Tapping:

Side of Hand: Even though I still feel afraid when I think of what happened, I deeply and completely love and accept myself anyway. Even though I can still feel the fear in my body, I deeply and completely love and accept myself now.

Eyebrow: My body remembers the fear.
Side of Eye: I feel afraid when I think about what happened.
Under Eye: I'm still afraid inside my body.
Under Nose: When I remember what happened, I feel scared.
Chin: I still feel afraid when I think of what happened.
Collarbone: I lived with fear all the time.
Under Arm: I still feel fearful all the time.
Head: I want to release this fear.

Take a deep breath, and use the 0-10 point scale to measure how that same memory of fear feels in your body. You can tweak the words I'm suggesting if that would be more accurate for your situation.

Side of Hand: Even though I can still bring up that fear when I think of what happened, I deeply and completely love and accept myself. Even though I lived in fear all the time, I accept who I am and how I feel.

Eyebrow: I lived with fear all the time.
Side of Eye: Specific memories bring up that fear now.
Under Eye: I can remember how afraid I was all the time.
Under Nose: I remember all my fear from my childhood.
Chin: It didn't really go anywhere.
Collarbone: I still feel afraid when I remember what happened.

Under Arm: I can recall my fear easily.
Head: I still feel the fear in my body.

Take another deep breath, and measure your fear now on the 0-10 point scale. You can recall any incident you felt afraid of in your childhood, or use the Tapping for something you're afraid of now as well. Proceed to the Gratitude Tapping.

Side of Hand: Even though I know I'm storing fear in my nervous system, I deeply and completely love and accept myself anyway. Even though I still have so much fear stored in my nervous system, I accept who I am and how I feel.
Eyebrow: I feel very grateful in spite of my fear.
Side of Eye: I have a lot to appreciate in my life.
Under Eye: I feel so grateful for so much in my life.
Under Nose: Thank you, Universe, for bringing me such joy.
Chin: I love feeling so grateful.
Collarbone: I appreciate so much about my life.
Under Arm: Thank you, Universe, for helping me feel so grateful.
Head: I choose to feel grateful every day.

Take a final deep breath and use the 0-10 point scale to measure the fear about that particular event or memory, or the general fear in your body, and continue using Tapping on your daily fear and anxiety.

Some people feel more anxiety than fear. If this is the case, go ahead and reword the sentences for the Tapping, and insert the phrase, "Even though I feel so anxious that something bad could happen…"

Betrayal

The final emotion I'm going to offer Tapping Sequences for is betrayal. So many people harbor feelings of betrayal in their current life because of something that happened in their childhood. Maybe a parent or sibling, neighbor, grandparent, friend, teacher, or coach betrayed you – or that's how you took it at the time – and you have the option now to tap on it and release it. This won't change what happened, but it will lighten the load in your emotional container, paving the way for more peace and contentment in your life.

Tapping Target: Betrayal

Think of a time you felt betrayed by someone in your life. Bring the person to mind, and the memory of when you "found out" what happened or what the betrayal was for you. On the 0-10 point scale, how high is the feeling of upset now? Proceed to the Tapping.

Side of Hand: Even though I felt so betrayed back then, I deeply and completely love and accept myself anyway. Even though I was so betrayed back then, and I can still feel it now, I accept who I am and how I feel.

Eyebrow: I remember feeling betrayed.
Side of Eye: My body remembers it too.
Under Eye: I remember being betrayed.
Under Nose: What an awful feeling.
Chin: I felt so betrayed when it happened.
Collarbone: I felt so betrayed back then.
Under Arm: I felt so betrayed.
Head: I can still feel it now.

Take a deep breath, think of the betrayal, and measure your stress or upset on the 0-10 point scale again. It should have decreased somewhat with this Tapping Round. If you need to tweak the wording to suit your situation, do that for this next round. When we feel betrayed, we often feel shocked, and the incident registers as a "trauma" in our bodies.

Side of Hand: Even though I still feel betrayed by what happened, and I was so surprised by it, I accept who I am and how I feel. Even though I still feel a sense of betrayal, I accept who I am and how I am feeling.

Eyebrow: I still feel betrayed by what happened.
Side of Eye: I remember the shock.
Under Eye: I still feel betrayed by what happened.
Under Nose: I still feel the shock in my body.

Chin: I was so surprised and shocked.
Collarbone: I still feel betrayed.
Under Arm: I still feel the betrayal.
Head: I feel sad about the betrayal.

Take another deep breath, and measure the feeling of betrayal again on the 0-10 point scale. Proceed to the Gratitude Tapping.

Side of Hand: Even though I still feel betrayed by what happened, I'm going to consider letting it go. Even though I can still feel the sting of being betrayed by what happened, I accept who I am now.
Eyebrow: I feel grateful anyway.
Side of Eye: I feel so grateful anyway.
Under Eye: Thank you, Universe, for showing me how far I've come.
Under Nose: Thank you, Universe, for the resolution about this.
Chin: I appreciate how much I've changed.
Collarbone: I appreciate all the lessons in my life.
Under Arm: I even appreciate most of my childhood.
Head: I feel grateful for so much in my life.

Take a final deep breath and measure this memory or feeling of betrayal on the 0-10 point scale. If you have several incidents that come to mind when you think of being betrayed, you may repeat these Tapping Sequences for each one, adjusting the wording to suit your real feelings.

There are many more emotions, memories, and conflicts we could tap on from childhood – feelings of resentment, impatience, regret, terror – the list could be endless. Choose which memories or feelings you'd like to work on, get specific about what your target phrase would sound like, and devise your own Tapping Scripts. Here are some more examples of memories or feelings that might be clogging your container:

- Even though I feel so resentful that I didn't get on the soccer team...
- Even though I feel so hurt about what they said behind my back...

- Even though I remember being teased in school…
- Even though I remember the teacher blaming me…
- Even though my father said I was _____…
- Even though my mother said I was too _____…

Now let's move on to the second big block that gets in the way of good self-care and sticking to a consistent gratitude practice; low self-esteem.

CHAPTER 6
Low Self-Esteem

Psychology Today estimated that 85% of people suffer from low self-esteem.[27] This means that they lack confidence in their abilities and don't feel a sense of worthiness, in spite of their accomplishments, skills, or character. If you suffer from low self-esteem, it will definitely be one of the biggest challenges blocking your ability to expand your capacity for more joy and happiness by using a gratitude practice.

For me, the second biggest block to my expanding my container for joy and happiness, after my preoccupation with the chaos in my family, was that my parents' alcoholism and repeated relapsing led to my feeling devalued. I suffered from low self-esteem and behaved as if I didn't deserve to take care of myself. I repeatedly neglected my emotional and physical self-care by putting the needs of others first, not standing up for myself, and overworking. While the symptoms of low self-esteem fall on a continuum, there are general qualities people with low self-esteem have in common. They don't value themselves, which means they have trouble setting good boundaries. They feel guilty when they say no because they don't want to disappoint anyone. They feel uncomfortable putting themselves first and spend way too much time and attention attending to other people's needs rather than focusing on habits or ways to improve their own lives. These symptoms reinforce their lack of value, perpetuating the cycle of *"I'm just not worth the trouble."*

I'll address four common symptoms or behavioral manifestations of low self-esteem and provide Tapping Sequences for each one.

1. Fear of saying no
2. Guilt when setting boundaries
3. Feeling inadequate
4. Neglecting self-care

Tapping Target: Low Self-Esteem

Before we use Tapping on the specific behavioral symptoms of low self-esteem, let's dig deeper into the actual cause of low self-esteem – how you developed your worth by seeing it reflected in your caretakers' words and actions.

We need to look at why you devalue yourself – what led you to believe you aren't valued? What was said to you? What did you hear or feel about yourself reflected in your caretakers' words, looks, behaviors, or feelings? What actually caused the low self-esteem in the first place? How we interpret our caretakers' messages about who we are and what we're worth is a pivotal piece in formulating self-esteem. Your memory of "what they said about me" or "what they did" definitely shaped your self-esteem.

In my case, my parents chose alcohol over me at an age where all kids need age appropriate validation, mirroring, boundaries, and affirmation. I knew they loved me, but I often felt devalued before my psyche was mature enough to understand their drinking behavior wasn't about me. I had to learn that it wasn't my fault, and that I didn't cause any of it.

Consider an attitude, a behavior, or a comment someone said to you that made you feel inadequate or devalued as a child. It's likely it didn't just happen once, but was a repeated occurrence in your life, leading to low self-esteem.

What do you remember being said about you that might have led you to believe you weren't valued? Remember that comment (or behavior), and see if you can give the memory a number on the 0-10 point scale. This number would represent the pain you feel when you think about it. For this Tapping Sequence, we'll use the target: *He said I wouldn't amount to anything.* You can substitute your own memory of what was said about you or done to you that may have informed your low self-esteem.

Side of Hand: Even though I remember what he said about me, that I wouldn't amount to anything, I deeply and completely love and accept myself anyway. Even though I distinctly remember him saying I would never amount to anything, I accept who I was back then and who I am now.

Eyebrow: I remember what he said about me.
Side of Eye: It still stings.
Under Eye: I never felt good enough.
Under Nose: He said I would never amount to anything.
Chin: I always felt dismissed.
Collarbone: I always tried to amount to something.
Under Arm: I never got his approval.
Head: I assumed I wasn't good enough.

Take a deep breath, and with that memory in mind, see if you can rate your distress again about this memory on the 0-10 point scale, and continue:

Side of Hand: Even though I'll never forget what he said about me, I accept who I am and how I feel about myself. Even though I have never felt like I measured up, and I've been trying hard my whole life, I choose to remember that his comment wasn't really about me.

Eyebrow: I still feel like I'm lacking something.
Side of Eye: I remember him saying I wouldn't amount to anything.
Under Eye: I believed him at the time.
Under Nose: I believed I wasn't worthy.
Chin: I didn't believe I deserved time or attention.
Collarbone: I've always tried to get someone's approval.
Under Arm: I'm still looking for his approval.
Head: I don't think I've ever amounted to anything.

Take another deep breath, and see if you can measure your distress about the target comment made about you on the 0-10 point scale. If it has been reduced a few points from where you started, go ahead and proceed to the Gratitude Tapping.

Side of Hand: Even though I've suffered a lot in my life, I choose to remember I still feel grateful. Even though I went through a lot of pain in my life, I accept who I am and how I feel.

Eyebrow: I'm so grateful for my life.
Side of Eye: I'm grateful I no longer believe him.
Under Eye: I appreciate all the lessons I have learned.
Under Nose: I appreciate that he was misinformed.
Chin: Thank you, Universe, for showing me how to value myself now.
Collarbone: I'm so thankful for all the value I offer my loved ones.
Under Arm: Thank you for showing me that I don't need anyone's approval.
Head: Thank you for all the loving relationships in my life.

Take a final deep breath, and use the 0-10 point scale to measure how you feel about the comment that was made that undermined your confidence. You may use these Tapping Sequences on any comments, behaviors, or attitudes towards you that were ill-informed, wrong, or coming from a place of bitterness, immaturity, or insecurity.

Let's move on now to another important target that people with low self-esteem suffer from in their lives: the fear of saying no.

Tapping Target: Fear of Saying No

Jenny

Jenny told me she was afraid to stand up to her boyfriend because she was convinced saying "no" would trigger him into leaving. He had threatened to leave before, and she admitted she would rather have him around than take the risk of standing up to him. She said that intellectually she knew this was counterproductive – and that if saying no would trigger a break-up, then there wasn't a solid foundation to begin with. But she said her fear gripped her and she always caved in to whatever he wanted – from where they went to dinner, to when they had sex, to what they watched on TV.

When I asked Jenny how high her fear was on the 0-10 point scale, she said: "It's off the charts. You're not going to make me say no after I leave here are you?"

"Of course I'm not going to ask you to do something you're not ready to do," I said. But I led her through some Tapping Rounds to release the intense fear and tension in her body at the thought of standing up to her boyfriend. Jenny quickly calmed her deep fear and immediately understood this was related to her mother "threatening to leave" her family when she was young. Once she could unpack this trigger and use Tapping on it, she started practicing saying no to her boyfriend in very small ways. She was still uncomfortable, but made good progress.

During one of her "practice" sessions of saying no, her boyfriend actually threatened to leave again. She kept quiet and didn't argue. Eventually he backed off his threat, but it gave her the information she needed: while he had great qualities, if this dynamic didn't change, there was no future for them. She started a gratitude practice about her value and what she liked about the relationship, and started to feel more comfortable in her body, saying no, and standing up to him. She had made tremendous progress by the time she ended therapy, and left with a list of where else she could use the Tapping to reduce her fears in her life. I heard from her a few months later. She informed me that while her behavior had changed, her boyfriend repeatedly threatened to leave whenever she stood up for herself, so she made the decision to end the relationship.

Imagine **saying no** in a situation you're facing right now at work or at home. You may feel afraid to say no because if you do, something bad will happen.

Measure your level of fear on the 0-10 point scale. Proceed to the Tapping Sequences I have written out for you.

Side of Hand: Even though I'm afraid to say no, I don't want to disappoint anyone, I deeply and completely love and accept myself anyway. Even though I'm afraid to say no, I accept who I am and how I feel.

Eyebrow: I'm afraid to say no.
Side of Eye: I don't want to say no.
Under Eye: I'm not sure I even know how to say no.
Under Nose: It makes me feel so uncomfortable.
Chin: I don't want to say no.
Collarbone: I don't want to hurt someone else.
Under Arm: I don't feel right when I put my needs first.
Head: I'm afraid to say no.

Take a deep breath, and measure your fear of saying no in that same situation on the 0-10 point scale.

Side of Hand: Even though I'm still afraid of saying no, what if I get rejected, I accept who I am and how I feel. Even though I'm still afraid of saying no, what if they get mad at me, I accept who I am and how I feel.

Eyebrow: I feel so stressed out.
Side of Eye: I have so much stress in my life.
Under Eye: I have so much stress everywhere.
Under Nose: I am very stressed out.
Chin: I'm not handling my stress very well.
Collarbone: I wish I didn't react so much.
Under Arm: I feel so much stress every day.
Head: I feel stress in every part of my life.

Take a deep breath, and measure your fear of saying no in the same situation again on the 0-10 point scale. You may keep Tapping on the original fear you tuned in to, or apply these sequences to a second or third situation until your comfort level with saying no increases dramatically. Proceed to the Gratitude Tapping below.

Side of Hand: Even though I'm still afraid to say no, I appreciate who I am and that I'm doing the best I can. Even though I'm still afraid to say no because I'm worried about their reactions, I accept who I am and how I feel about it.

Eyebrow: I appreciate that I'm doing the best I can.
Side of Eye: I'm so thankful that I feel better.
Under Eye: Thank you, Universe, for so many blessings.
Under Nose: I have so much to appreciate in my life.
Chin: Thank you, Universe, for so many blessings in my life.
Collarbone: Thank you, Universe, for all the wisdom about saying no.
Under Arm: I'm so thankful that I've improved my self-esteem.
Head: I appreciate how much I've changed.

Take a final deep breath, and measure how afraid you feel now of saying no in the situation you chose for your original target. You may apply these Tapping Sequences to other situations where you feel uncomfortable saying no, and tap until your feelings decrease and you find yourself willing to say no and stand up for yourself more often. Even a slight decrease in the discomfort and fear will change your behavior with others.

Tapping Target: Guilt About Setting Boundaries

The second prevalent symptom or result of suffering from low self-esteem that we can target with Tapping, is feeling guilty when we try to set clear boundaries in order to take care of ourselves and our needs. You either feel guilty and selfish, or you're afraid someone else will *accuse you* of being selfish. Putting yourself first triggers feelings of anxiety that someone might get mad at you.

Marion

Marion came to me because of her physical and emotional exhaustion. Her friend who had witnessed her avoiding setting boundaries with family members referred her to me for Tapping. Marion's description of the problem was that she was overworked, didn't get enough sleep, and was eating a poor diet. When I asked why her friend had referred her to a Tapping therapist, she wasn't sure. "She said something about my inability to set boundaries, but I don't think that's the problem." As the session unfolded, it became crystal clear that guilt ran Marion's behavior. She was a self-described people-pleaser and felt guilty whenever she wanted to set a time boundary with anyone at work or at home. "But wouldn't that be unkind of me?" She was even the go-to neighborhood driver for carpooling kids to soccer when their parents needed an extra hand.

When I asked Marion why she didn't set more boundaries more often, she just shrugged her shoulders and said: "I think it's mean when I have the time and can chip in." When I reminded her that she had sought help because she was exhausted and burned out, she reconsidered the value of setting boundaries in every area of her life. When I asked her why she thought she had so much guilt, she immediately knew that her mother had modeled this behavior, and even guilted her and her siblings when they said they didn't have the time to help out extended family members. After a lot of Tapping and releasing, Marion started to feel physically restored and more mentally rested. This gave her the emotional strength to set boundaries with her family and neighbors, even when she thought she was being unreasonable. Eventually, setting better boundaries allowed her to start making more space for herself, including her hobbies, her needs, deep rest, and even a gratitude practice.

Consider setting a specific boundary with a friend, colleague or family member, and measure how guilty you feel now on the 0-10 point scale. Try this Tapping Sequence on your guilt about taking care of yourself with good boundaries.

Side of Hand: Even though I feel guilty whenever I try to set good boundaries, I accept who I am and how I feel anyway. Even though I always feel guilty when I try to put myself first and set a boundary with others, I deeply and completely love and accept who I am.

Eyebrow: I cringe when I have to set a boundary.
Side of Eye: I know I need to set better boundaries.
Under Eye: It makes me feel too guilty.
Under Nose: I feel guilty when I set boundaries.
Chin: When I feel guilty, I back down.

Collarbone: It's hard to stand up for myself.
Under Arm: I usually back down.
Head: I feel too guilty setting boundaries.

Take a deep breath, and tune back in to the discomfort you originally felt when thinking of setting a specific boundary with a friend, colleague, or family member. Measure how guilty you feel now on the 0-10 point scale. Continue with the following Tapping Round:

Side of Hand: Even though it's hard for me to set clear boundaries, I end up feeling guilty, I deeply and completely love and accept myself anyway. Even though I still feel guilty when I set boundaries, I accept who I am and how I feel.

Eyebrow: I still feel guilty when I need to set a boundary.
Side of Eye: I still feel so guilty setting boundaries.
Under Eye: I want to take care of myself.
Under Nose: But I always put them first.
Chin: I feel so guilty setting boundaries.
Collarbone: I still feel guilty setting boundaries.
Under Arm: I don't think I'm allowed to set boundaries.
Head: I don't value myself enough to set a boundary.

Take another deep breath, and while tuning in to the scenario of setting a boundary with the original person you imagined, measure your guilt now on the 0-10 point scale. You can repeat these Tapping Rounds again for different scenarios in your life, or move on to the Gratitude Tapping below.

Side of Hand: Even though I still feel guilty whenever I try to set boundaries, I deeply and completely love and accept myself anyway. Even though I still struggle with guilt because I don't think I'm worth the trouble to set boundaries, I choose to appreciate how much progress I've made.

Eyebrow: I feel guilty but I'm grateful for this opportunity.
Side of Eye: Thank you, Universe, for showing me my value.
Under Eye: I've decided to appreciate myself anyway.
Under Nose: There is so much to appreciate about myself.

Chin: Thank you, Universe, for helping me set good boundaries.
Collarbone: Thank you for showing me that I'm worth it.
Under Arm: Thank you, Universe, for helping me appreciate my worth.
Head: Thank you for showing me my value.

Take another deep breath, and measure your guilt now on the 0-10 point scale. You may continue using Tapping on your guilt about setting boundaries with anyone in your life. Some of your target statements might sound like: "It doesn't feel right to set a boundary" or "They'll get mad at me" or "I was taught it was selfish to set boundaries." When you're ready, proceed to the next symptom of suffering with low self-esteem.

Tapping Target: Feeling Inadequate/Not Enough

An additional cause of low self-esteem is the entrenched belief that you are deeply inadequate. You never assess yourself as being enough on any level – your skill set, your loyalty, your intelligence, or who you are at your core. Your accomplishments rarely make a dent in this low assessment of yourself.

You don't believe in yourself or believe that you are capable of finishing what you set out to accomplish. And even when you do, you second guess your results. This cycle is mentally exhausting and digs you into a deeper hole every time you question your value.

Measure how "adequate" you feel on the 0-10 point scale right now. Maybe you need to picture yourself in a relationship, a work scenario, or in a friendship. Do you think you're "enough" and that your attributes are valuable? It's challenging to evaluate what you think your worth is, but see if you can get a sense of where you land on the measurement scale.

Another way to approach the measurement is to ask yourself how true "I feel inadequate" feels on the 0-10 point scale. Start Tapping for this adequacy/worthiness issue.

Side of Hand: Even though I'm convinced I'm inadequate and don't have what it takes to be successful, I accept who I am and how I feel. Even though I don't believe in myself and my worth, I accept who I am and how I feel.

Eyebrow: I've never believed I had what it takes.
Side of Eye: I don't have what it takes because I'm inadequate.
Under Eye: I don't believe in myself or my skills.
Under Nose: I don't value myself; I'm just not enough.
Chin: I'm not adequate and never have been.
Collarbone: I've never been adequate.
Under Arm: I don't believe in myself and never have.
Head: I don't believe I have what it takes.

Take a deep breath and measure how true this statement about being inadequate still feels on the 0-10 point scale. Continue:

Side of Hand: Even though I still feel inadequate, I never measure up, I deeply and completely love and accept who I am and how I feel. Even though I still feel deeply inadequate, I accept who I am and how I feel.

Eyebrow: I still feel inadequate.
Side of Eye: I've always felt inadequate.
Under Eye: I've never thought I was enough.
Under Nose: I'm convinced I don't measure up.
Chin: I've never been enough.
Collarbone: And I'm still not enough.
Under Arm: I still feel dissatisfied with myself.
Head: I am still convinced that I'll never measure up.

Take another deep breath and see if you can measure any changes in your belief about yourself on the 0-10 point scale. Sometimes after Tapping, the feeling of inadequacy won't feel as strong, or you'll feel more neutral about the topic of your value. You'll think it's *less true* that you don't measure up. You can keep using Tapping on the above sequences to increase your assessment that you are enough, or move to the Gratitude Tapping below.

Side of Hand: Even though I still feel inadequate and always have, I accept that I feel better and stronger now. Even though I've always felt that I wasn't enough, I accept who I am and how I feel now.

Eyebrow: I'm so grateful for who I am.

Side of Eye: I appreciate who I've become.

Under Eye: I appreciate how hard I've struggled.

Under Nose: I'm so grateful that I know my value.

Chin: Thank you, Universe, for showing me how to appreciate my value.

Collarbone: I value myself and am grateful for who I am.

Under Arm: Thank you, Universe, for all my new insights.

Head: Thank you for who I've become.

Take a final deep breath and measure how true this belief feels to you now on the 0-10 point scale. You may repeat these sequences whenever you see your behavior reflect a sense of inadequacy in your life. The more you release this belief, the more your behavior will reflect a person who appreciates their worth.

Tapping Target: Neglecting Self-Care

Doing more for others at the expense of your own needs isn't healthy for anyone. If you don't put the oxygen mask on yourself first, you won't be emotionally available to help others anyway. For this exercise, you could measure your discomfort at putting yourself first on the 0-10 point scale, or measure the stress of feeling like a selfish person when you focus on your own needs. When either of these two feelings are neutralized, you will start to take better care of yourself and your needs.

Go ahead and use the 0-10 point scale to measure your discomfort when you think of putting yourself first. You may need to tune in to a particular relationship to feel the emotional charge.

Side of Hand: Even though I feel so uncomfortable putting my needs first, I deeply and completely love and accept myself anyway. Even though I feel such discomfort at the thought of taking care of myself, I accept who I am and how I feel.

Eyebrow: I feel so uncomfortable putting my needs first.
Side of Eye: It feels so awkward.
Under Eye: It feels selfish.
Under Nose: I'm worried I'll be called selfish.
Chin: It feels so unnatural to put myself first.
Collarbone: I don't think I deserve it.
Under Arm: I think they should come first.
Head: It's hard to put my needs first.

Take a deep breath, and measure that feeling of discomfort as you imagine putting yourself first on the 0-10 point scale. Continue:

Side of Hand: Even though I still feel awkward and uncomfortable when I put my needs first, I deeply and completely love and accept myself anyway. Even though it doesn't feel right when I focus on myself, I accept who I am and how I feel.
Eyebrow: It feels so awkward when I put my needs first.
Side of Eye: It doesn't feel right.
Under Eye: It doesn't feel normal.
Under Nose: I'm used to taking care of someone else.
Chin: I'm worried I'll be called selfish.
Collarbone: I'm worried I am being selfish.
Under Arm: It still feels so awkward to put myself first.
Head: I feel so uncomfortable putting myself first.

Take another deep breath and use the 0-10 point scale to measure how awkward or uncomfortable it feels in the situation you imagined. Proceed to the Gratitude Tapping below.

Side of Hand: Even though it feels too uncomfortable to put myself first, I deeply and completely love and accept myself anyway. Even though I'm convinced I'm going to be called selfish, I accept who I am and how I feel.
Eyebrow: I appreciate the needs I have.
Side of Eye: I'm ready to appreciate myself and my needs.
Under Eye: I really feel grateful for who I am.

Under Nose: I'm grateful that I value myself more and more.
Chin: Thank you, Universe, for bringing me all my gifts.
Collarbone: Thank you, Universe, for all the lessons I have learned.
Under Arm: Thank you, Universe, for so many valuable insights.
Head: I'm so thankful for who I am.

Take a final deep breath, and measure your discomfort again on the 0-10 point scale. You may continue using Tapping on any variations of this theme until you start to see your behavior change. It may still feel awkward when you put yourself first, but you will notice and appreciate the new ways you value yourself and your own needs.

Tapping Target: There Won't Be Enough For Me

Now let's address a common problem related to the issue of low self-esteem. In addition to feeling as if you're *not enough*, many people with low self-esteem are convinced that *there won't be enough for them*.

Do you believe this – that there won't be enough for you? Enough food, money, love, or anything you want? This is called "scarcity consciousness". Usually, you learn it from your experiences as a child. But even when your situation changes, the feelings and beliefs remain in the shadows.

Carrie

Carrie was the 4th of 7 kids in her family, and she said she was definitely "the forgotten middle child." She was embarrassed to tell me she hoarded money. It didn't matter how much she had, she never let go of any of it. It was an extreme reaction to her childhood of poverty. When I asked her to give me some examples of how she learned about poverty, she said her mother always had to use the same teabag 3 times, they could never throw anything out, and the kids were always hungry and asking for more snacks. She said their school lunches were too small, and there was never anything in the refrigerator when they got home from school. Carrie was mortified by her hand-me-downs, and never had anyone over after school because the house was so rundown. Her parents constantly said, "There's not enough for all of us, so we have to make do."

Carrie was convinced this was tied to her value and her self-esteem. When she used Tapping on her fear that there wouldn't be enough, and the belief that she wasn't "worth" giving to, she dramatically changed this feeling of scarcity. She was eventually able to stick to her gratitude practice and tune in to how much her friends valued her and how much value she had in her life.

The belief that there won't be enough for you may have come from your childhood, but you can swap out this belief for a healthier, more positive one. Try this Tapping Sequence below.

Measure how true this belief feels to you on the 0-10 point scale – *I'm convinced there will never be enough for me.*

Side of Hand: Even though I'm convinced there will never be enough for me, there never has been, I deeply and completely love and accept myself. Even though I'm convinced there will never be enough for me, I accept where I learned this and how I feel about it.

Eyebrow: There will never be enough for me.
Side of Eye: There never was enough for me.
Under Eye: I'm sure there never will be enough.
Under Nose: I think it's because I'm not enough.
Chin: I'm tired of it, but it's my fault.
Collarbone: But I'm convinced it won't change.
Under Arm: There will never be enough for me.
Head: There never was and there never will be.

Take a deep breath, and measure how true this belief feels to you now on the 0-10 point scale. If a particular memory surfaces for you, go ahead and do a Tapping Round on that memory as well. Evaluate the distress you feel when you remember what happened, and go ahead and use Tapping on the feelings.

Side of Hand: Even though I'm still convinced there will never be enough for me, that's how it's always been, I accept who I am and how I feel. Even though I'm still convinced there will never be enough for me, I deeply and profoundly love and accept myself anyway.

Eyebrow: I'm still convinced there won't be enough for me.
Side of Eye: There never has been enough.
Under Eye: Why would anything change?
Under Nose: There has never been enough for me.
Chin: I don't expect there ever to be enough.
Collarbone: I've never been enough.
Under Arm: There will never be enough of what I need.
Head: I'm still convinced there will never be enough for me.

Take another deep breath, and measure how true this belief feels to you now on the 0-10 point scale. Proceed to the Gratitude Tapping below.

Side of Hand: Even though there's never been enough for me, I'm willing to expect things to change. Even though there's never been enough for me, I'm grateful for all the benefits I have in my life now.

Eyebrow: I'm so grateful for all of my abundance.
Side of Eye: Thank you, Universe, for bringing me so much abundance.
Under Eye: I'm grateful for the abundance I have in my life.
Under Nose: Thank you for all the abundance I enjoy.
Chin: I love feeling grateful for what I enjoy in my life.
Collarbone: Thank you, Universe, for bringing me so many blessings.
Under Arm: I appreciate the abundance I notice in my life.
Head: I love and appreciate so much abundance in my life.

Take a final deep breath and measure how true this original belief – *there is never enough for me* – feels to you now on the 0-10 point scale.

Now let's move on to clearing the final block to living your best life – self-sabotaging behavior, and the feelings and beliefs that drive it.

CHAPTER 7
Self-Sabotaging Behavior

Self-sabotaging behavior is the third block to keeping a consistent gratitude practice. These behaviors include procrastination, perfectionism, people-pleasing, addictions, and generally, anything you do that blocks your forward movement. These behaviors keep us from consistently sticking to routines and habits that are good for us, including keeping a gratitude practice.

The key question is: why would you sabotage yourself? The answer is: to keep yourself from feeling better, standing out, or shining. When you stay small, you can't be a target for anyone else's conflicts about your emotional, physical, financial, or professional success.

All your self-sabotaging behaviors stem from a fear of success or a fear of failure. We use self-sabotaging behavior to protect us, keep us small, safe, and invisible, so we don't become a target. If you're afraid of success, you don't want to stand out and be a target of someone's jealousy. We know that sticking to a gratitude practice will definitely make you more successful, happy, healthy, and peaceful. And if you feel the need to avoid feeling better to stay safe, you'll choose one of the many self-sabotaging patterns to get in your own way.

If you're afraid of failure, you also don't want to be seen and will use self-sabotaging behavior so you don't stand out and get criticized, or judged as a fraud or imposter. When you're afraid of failure, you don't naturally lean towards a self-care practice as impressive as the superpower of gratitude. You're too busy protecting yourself. You are risk averse, and feel safer playing small and under the radar. *You are not focused on feeling better; you're focused on surviving.*

It may be confusing to understand why people would put a lid on their success and happiness. But if being happier feels threatening to you because of other people's reactions, you'll move heaven and earth to stay invisible, and you certainly won't want to take advantage of using a superpower as promising as gratitude.

Remember our discussion in Part 2 about the positive intent of self-sabotaging behavior – you're only trying to protect yourself from something you fear. You're actually trying to keep yourself feeling emotionally safe. Dramatically improving your health, life, relationships, and happiness with gratitude would definitely raise a red flag because it would make you shine and be more visible. Remember, self-sabotaging behavior is about staying invisible. Once you ask the right questions and get the answers clearly categorized into fears and beliefs, you'll be able to translate them into effective EFT Tapping setup phrases for your healing.

Fear of Success and Fear of Failure

In order to expand your capacity for more joy and happiness, you're going to need to address your fear of success and your fear of failure, since these fears trigger most of your protective behavior. These major fears might manifest as different behaviors, but they are both driven by intense emotions and limiting beliefs that are keeping you hiding under the radar.

If you are unable to resolve these fears, you will stay stuck in the cycle of sabotaging your efforts to move forward personally or professionally. In addition, you won't be compelled to reach for more tools to make yourself feel better.

If you're afraid of success, you'll dismiss the success you already have in your life and try to stay hidden under the radar. You won't want to be a target for someone else and you won't want your success to be taken away once you have it.

If you're afraid of failure, you will be in a constant state of fear and won't feel interested in looking for things to appreciate. You will avoid completing projects, and you won't be able to stick to your practices that make you feel better, no matter what the costs. The risk of your happiness being yanked away once you have it is too threatening.

Fear of Success

Are you afraid to be more successful, joyful, content, and happy than you already are? Might this be the answer to the "upside" of staying stuck? If you are afraid to be successful, you could ask yourself the upside/downside questions again, or refer back to your answers to the questions I listed in Chapter 3 to understand the real fears and beliefs that keep you playing small.

- What is the upside to staying stuck?
- What is the downside of reaching your goals?

There are many reasons people feel *afraid to succeed*. From my 30 plus years of experience as a psychotherapist, these are the most common reasons clients are afraid of success:

- Fear of having success and happiness taken away.
- Fear of being visible/shining/standing out.
- Fear of being a target of other people's jealousy.
- Fear of other people's expectations.

There are also many limiting beliefs that block people from being more successful. Common beliefs that block your success might be:

- Being successful is unsafe for me.
- I believe in struggle and hardship.
- I don't have what it takes to be more successful.
- I'm convinced it's too late, so why bother trying.

Whether you struggle with fears, or beliefs that are stopping your forward momentum, you will likely convert these emotions and beliefs into self-sabotaging behaviors that stop you in your tracks. Whether you procrastinate, show up late, pick a fight, or use excuses to hold yourself back, all the behaviors protect you from moving forward in order to satisfy the *upside of staying the same*. They have a protective purpose to keep you emotionally safe.

If your fear of success stems from the fear of being visible, you will likely block your success at work and at home, as well as "forget" to stick to your gratitude practice. The result? You get to stay under the radar, play small, and don't have to stretch your capacity for more joy and happiness. You'll feel emotionally safe, but likely dissatisfied.

> *Do you know why you're afraid of being successful, and therefore, more visible?*

It's likely that you have a part of you that wants to shine, stand out, and feel more joy and contentment, and another part of you that is protecting you because of something that happened in the past that you are trying to avoid. That's the reason for getting in your own way; you are consciously or unconsciously trying to keep yourself safe. Below I will offer Tapping Scripts for several of the fears and beliefs under the topics of Fear of Success and Fear of Failure.

Patsy

Patsy talked constantly about how she wanted to be more successful, make more money, and have more freedom in her work schedule. Yet every time she set out to advance her skills and position at work, she collapsed and did something to block her forward momentum. She would catch a virus, sprain an ankle, pick a fight with her partner, or say something inappropriate to her boss. She sought help from me after a self-sabotaging incident where she was sarcastic towards her boss in front of her colleagues. He sent her to Human Resources, who sent her to me for an evaluation.

The reason she was getting in her own way became obvious when I asked her to question her own motives. "What might be the upside to sabotaging your success and staying stuck?" She picked at her pink manicure and said, "then I'll be criticized by the others." While she had a dream of advancing at work, she could feel the jealousy of the all-female staff with a male boss. "When did this happen to you before?" She admitted that in High School she had stood out in drama class, was given the biggest role in the school play, and was accused of sleeping with the drama teacher, even by her closest friends. She said the accusations devastated her, but she hid her feelings and just told them to "F off." Nothing had happened with the teacher. She got the part because of her vocal range and ability to dance. She admitted she developed a fear of success because she was afraid that the joy would be ruined again. After careful consideration, she theorized that she had been sabotaging her success ever since that event.

Once this pattern was uncovered, I taught her how to use Tapping on the memory of the event, the hurt she had felt from her friends' accusations, and on her fear of standing out again. She started a regular gratitude practice, learned to appreciate her challenges and her experiences, and was able to make steady progress with clear boundaries at work.

Tapping Target: Fear of Success Being Taken Away

Think of reaching the next level of personal or professional success. Can you feel the risk of it being yanked away from you? This would naturally feel like anxiety or fear. Maybe you could imagine feeling happier and more joyful, but then anticipate that it could be taken away from you. See if you can measure this fear of your success, however you define it, being taken away from you on the 0-10 point scale.

Side of Hand: Even though I'm afraid to be happier and more successful because it might be taken away from me, I deeply and completely love and accept myself anyway. Even though I'm afraid to be more joyful and successful because it might be taken away from me, I accept who I am and how I feel about this.

Eyebrow: I'm afraid to be more successful.
Side of Eye: What if it gets taken away from me?
Under Eye: I'm afraid to lose it once I have it.

Under Nose: I'm afraid to feel much better.
Chin: I don't want to lose it again.
Collarbone: I'm afraid to lose it once I have it.
Under Arm: What if it gets taken away from me?
Head: No wonder I sabotage my success and happiness.

Take a deep breath, and measure this fear again on the 0-10 point scale. If any memories surface from another time in your life when this happened, write down the details and use that memory for another Tapping Sequence after this one.

Side of Hand: Even though I'm still afraid of being happier and more successful because of the risk it could be taken away from me, I deeply and completely love and accept myself anyway. Even though I'm still afraid of getting what I want because then it could be taken away, I accept who I am and how I feel.
Eyebrow: I'm still afraid of being more successful.
Side of Eye: If I'm happier, they might take it away.
Under Eye: Feeling good doesn't last.
Under Nose: I'm afraid of feeling better, it might be taken away.
Chin: No wonder I sabotage myself.
Collarbone: I don't want it to be taken away.
Under Arm: No wonder I get in my own way.
Head: I'm afraid I'll lose what I have once I get it.

Take another deep breath, and measure this fear of your happiness and success being taken away from you on the 0-10 point scale. Proceed to the Gratitude Tapping.

Side of Hand: Even though I'm afraid to get what I want because it might be taken away, I deeply and completely love and accept myself. Even though I'm afraid to get what I want because it might be taken away from me, I accept who I am and where this came from.
Eyebrow: I'm grateful for the success I have.
Side of Eye: I appreciate all the happiness I have.

Under Eye: Thank you, Universe, for such a beautiful life.
Under Nose: Thank you, Universe, for all the blessings I enjoy.
Chin: Thank you, Universe, for showing me so much abundance.
Collarbone: Thank you for showing me how to take the risk.
Under Arm: Thank you, Universe, for so much to appreciate.
Head: I'm thankful for everything in my life right now.

Take a final deep breath, and measure this fear again on the 0-10 point scale. You may want to tune in to a specific incident or memory of a time when your success was suddenly taken away from you. Be specific with the wording, and start a new Tapping Sequence.

Tapping Target: Fear of Shining/Being Visible

First, measure how afraid you are of being visible, shining, or standing out on the 0-10 point scale. Maybe you'll tune in to a past event where standing out or shining got you into trouble or your success was suddenly ruined or taken away. Try this Tapping Sequence:

Side of Hand: Even though I'm afraid to shine and be more visible, what if they hurt me again, I deeply and completely love and accept myself. Even though I'm afraid to shine and be hurt again, I accept who I am and how I feel.

Eyebrow: It doesn't feel safe to shine.
Side of Eye: I don't want to stand out.
Under Eye: What if they pick on me?
Under Nose: I'm so anxious about shining.
Chin: No wonder I'm getting in my own way.
Collarbone: I'm worried about standing out.
Under Arm: It's not safe to be visible.
Head: I have mixed feelings about standing out.

Take a deep breath. Now measure your fear of shining and being visible again on the 0-10 point scale. Continue:

Side of Hand: Even though I'm still afraid to shine, I remember what happened last time, I deeply and completely love and accept myself anyway. Even though I'm still afraid to succeed, I might become a target, I accept who I am and how I feel about it.

Eyebrow: It doesn't feel safe to shine.
Side of Eye: I'm still afraid to shine.
Under Eye: I remember what happened last time.
Under Nose: I'm still worried about standing out.
Chin: No wonder I'm blocking my success.
Collarbone: I don't want to stand out.
Under Arm: It's not safe to be visible.
Head: It still doesn't feel safe to stand out.

Take another deep breath, and measure your fear of shining again on the 0-10 point scale. You may continue to tap on the fear of shining, standing out, and being visible, or proceed to the Gratitude Tapping below.

Side of Hand: Even though I'm still afraid to shine and be visible, I accept who I am and how I feel. Even though I'm still afraid to stand out and be visible, what if they hurt me again, I accept all of my feelings on this topic.

Eyebrow: Thank you, Universe, for connecting me to so much gratitude.
Side of Eye: I want to remember to feel grateful for my life.
Under Eye: I appreciate being grateful for my joy and success.
Under Nose: I appreciate how much I already shine.
Chin: I appreciate other people who shine.
Collarbone: Thank you, Universe, for so many opportunities.
Under Arm: Thank you for all my talents and skills.
Head: I'm so grateful for all the blessings I have in my life.

Take a final deep breath, and measure your fear of shining or being visible again on the 0-10 point scale. Continue Tapping until you've unpacked this fear of success and shining, or until you notice your behavior has changed and you no longer get in your own way. If you need to tune in to another incident from your past where you were happy and then suddenly something bad happened, replace the target with your own wording reflecting your experience.

Tapping Target: Fear of Their Expectations

A particular tension and pressure that builds for people who become more successful, is fearing other people's expectations. The result? You might procrastinate as a way to block your success, so you don't feel the pressure of their expectations of you. Is this a pressure or concern for you? See if you can measure your *fear of their expectations* on the 0-10 point scale. Start Tapping:

Side of Hand: Even though I'm afraid my success will increase their expectations of me, and I don't like the pressure, I accept who I am and how I feel. Even though I feel the pressure of having to maintain my success, I accept who I am and how I feel.

Eyebrow: I feel the pressure of their expectations.
Side of Eye: My success might trigger their expectations.
Under Eye: I'm afraid of the tension of their expectations.
Under Nose: I don't know how I'm going to manage it.
Chin: I don't want to have to manage their expectations.
Collarbone: I feel so much pressure about this.
Under Arm: No wonder I sabotage myself.
Head: No wonder I don't get anything done.

Take a deep breath and measure this fear of their expectations again on the 0-10 point scale and continue Tapping:

Side of Hand: Even though I'm still afraid they'll increase their expectations of me, I accept who I am and how I feel. Even though I'm still afraid my success will make them pressure me to do more, I accept who I am and how I feel.

Eyebrow: I'm afraid of their expectations.
Side of Eye: How will I maintain my success?
Under Eye: I don't want to feel their expectations.
Under Nose: I don't want to feel the pressure.

Chin: I can feel the pressure to keep succeeding.
Collarbone: I'm afraid of this tension.
Under Arm: No wonder I sabotage my success.
Head: It's just too much pressure.

Take a deep breath, and measure your fear of other people's expectations of you again on the 0-10 point scale. Proceed to the Gratitude Tapping.

Side of Hand: Even though I'm still afraid my success will make them pressure me to do even more, I deeply and completely love and accept myself anyway. Even though I'm still afraid of the pressure of their expectations, I accept all of me anyway.
Eyebrow: I appreciate my success already.
Side of Eye: I love feeling so satisfied about my success.
Under Eye: I'm grateful for the progress I've made.
Under Nose: Thank you, Universe, for all the progress I've made.
Chin: I'm grateful that I've come so far on this topic.
Collarbone: I appreciate all that I've learned.
Under Arm: I'm grateful for the lessons I've learned in my life.
Head: Thank you, Universe, for all the blessings I have in my life.

Take a final deep breath, and measure this fear again on the 0-10 point scale. If you feel you need to tap more on this fear to neutralize it more, go ahead and change the wording or address more specifically who "they" might be in your life who you fear might pressure you.

Tapping Target: Being Successful Is Unsafe

This target is clearly related to feeling afraid to shine and stand out, but we'll address it as a belief.

Sandra

Sandra entered therapy because she didn't like the direction her life was going. She was gaining weight, feeling more depressed, felt unappreciated at work, and was still locked into emotional battles with her sisters. She described herself as a hardcore pessimist and worrywart.

The youngest of 5 kids, Sandra felt she was always picked on by her siblings for being slow, lazy, sad, or watching too much television. At 45, she still felt like the family scapegoat. Sandra learned how to use Tapping for her heavy feelings associated with being uninspired and sad about her life. When she felt better, she was able to start a gratitude practice, which brightened her attitude and mood impressively. She didn't know anything about the amazing statistics, she just knew it made her feel a lot better in a short period of time. When her mood improved from the Tapping and her gratitude practice, she started spending more time outside, lost some extra weight, and was generally in a more playful mood. She said, "I still have the same unappreciative boss, but I feel much better." Sandra noticed that she was still a target for her siblings' criticism, but now they had to find new things to bug her about since she had lost weight and was much less apathetic than she used to be. Her siblings were clearly uncomfortable with her obvious emotional progress and happiness. They made fun of her new sunny disposition, said she was unrecognizable, and said her new mood was "unrealistic and wouldn't last".

Sandra said she was "stunned" that her siblings "would be so uncomfortable" with her newfound happiness. She fully believed that they preferred her personality when she expressed her worries all day long. After a few days of doubting whether withstanding the heat from her unhappy siblings was worth it, she got back on track with her new practice. She noticed improvements in her sleep, and decreased episodes of "swirling in negativity."

On the 0-10 point scale, how high is your belief that *being successful or happy is unsafe*? You may need to imagine yourself going to the next level professionally or personally to get an accurate reading on the measurement scale. Proceed to the Tapping Sequence for this limiting belief.

Side of Hand: Even though I'm convinced that being happier and more successful would be unsafe, I deeply and completely love and accept myself anyway. Even though I'm convinced that being happier and more successful would make me unsafe, I accept who I am and how I feel.

Eyebrow: I know that being much happier is unsafe.

Side of Eye: I remember what happened last time.
Under Eye: Being successful might be unsafe.
Under Nose: I remember how they treated me last time.
Chin: I don't believe I'm safe if I'm happy.
Collarbone: I'm convinced I would be unsafe.
Under Arm: Being successful and happy would be unsafe for me.
Head: No wonder I'm getting in my own way.

Take a deep breath, and measure how true this limiting belief feels to you now on the 0-10 point scale. You may need to tune in again to the image of you being more successful to get an accurate reading on the scale. Or you may need to tune in to what happened the "last time you were successful" to measure your fear of something bad happening again. Continue Tapping:

Side of Hand: Even though I still think being successful and happier will make me unsafe, I deeply and completely love and accept myself anyway. Even though I'm still convinced that being successful might put me in danger, I accept who I am and how I feel.
Eyebrow: I still feel unsafe when I'm happier.
Side of Eye: I'm still convinced being successful is unsafe.
Under Eye: I remember what happened last time.
Under Nose: I assume it will happen again.
Chin: I know I could be in danger again.
Collarbone: I don't want to feel unsafe again.
Under Arm: No wonder I hold myself back.
Head: I'm convinced it's unsafe to be happy and content.

Take another deep breath, and see if you can measure how true this belief feels to you now on the 0-10 point scale. Has it been neutralized at all? You may go back and use Tapping for the original issue that "taught" you this belief. When you feel ready, proceed to the Gratitude Tapping.

Side of Hand: Even though I'm still convinced that being successful and happier would make me unsafe, I deeply and completely love and accept myself anyway. Even though I'm still convinced it's safer to stay under the radar, I choose to appreciate the success I've already enjoyed.

Eyebrow: I appreciate my successes already.
Side of Eye: I'm so grateful for how far I've come.
Under Eye: Thank you, Universe, for all the support I have in my life.
Under Nose: Thank you for all my friends and colleagues.
Chin: Thank you for the emotional success I already enjoy.
Collarbone: I appreciate all the blessings in my life.
Under Arm: Thank you, Universe, for helping me feel safe.
Head: Thank you for all the blessings I have in my life.

Take a final deep breath, and see if you can measure the "truth" of the belief that being successful is unsafe on the 0-10 point scale. Keep Tapping until that belief has been neutralized and you feel confident about taking your next steps forward.

Tapping Target: I Believe in Struggle

A belief that will always block your success is the belief in struggle. Do you believe you need to struggle as a way of life, as a rite of passage, as a way of being? If so, you likely learned the "value" of struggle from people you care about or whom you admired. You may have learned that struggle was noble, and if you become successful, you'll be betraying this belief or value from your family. If you have this belief, you will most likely block your success by repeatedly making things harder for yourself, sabotaging your forward momentum.

Try to measure how true your belief in struggle is on the 0-10 point scale. Do you believe life has to be hard? Try this Tapping Sequence:

Side of Hand: Even though I'm convinced I need to struggle at work and at home, I think life has to be hard, I accept who I am and how I feel. Even though I'm convinced I need to struggle to fit in, I accept who I am and how I feel.

Eyebrow: I'm convinced I have to struggle.
Side of Eye: I won't fit in if I don't.

Under Eye: I'm convinced I have to struggle.
Under Nose: Doesn't everyone have to struggle?
Chin: It won't feel right if I don't struggle.
Collarbone: I want to fit in.
Under Arm: I'm convinced I have to struggle.
Head: Who would I be without my struggle?

Take a deep breath and measure how true your belief that you have to struggle is now, on the 0-10 point scale. Complete a second Tapping Round on this limiting belief.

Side of Hand: Even though I still believe I have to struggle, I accept who I am and how I feel. Even though I'm still convinced I have to struggle, I accept who I am and how I feel about this belief.
Eyebrow: I'm still convinced I have to struggle.
Side of Eye: I want to fit in.
Under Eye: Struggling still feels normal to me.
Under Nose: It still feels right to struggle.
Chin: It feels right to complain too.
Collarbone: I wonder if I could let this go.
Under Arm: I'm starting to get tired of struggling.
Head: I wonder what it would be like to let this go.

Take a deep breath, measure how true this belief feels to you now on the 0-10 point scale, and then proceed to the Gratitude Tapping.

Side of Hand: Even though I have always believed in struggle, it feels normal, I accept who I am and how I feel. Even though I've always struggled and don't see a way out of this, I accept who I am and where I learned this.
Eyebrow: I'm grateful for how hard I've worked.
Side of Eye: Thank you, Universe, for all the lessons I have learned.
Under Eye: Thank you, Universe, for how much I appreciate about my life.
Under Nose: I'm grateful knowing I can let go of the struggle.
Chin: I appreciate my desire to move on from this.

Collarbone: Thank you, Universe, for helping me let go of this struggle.
Under Arm: I appreciate that I'm ready to move on.
Head: Thank you for the lessons I've learned.

Take a final deep breath, measure your belief in struggle on the 0-10 point scale, and continue with the topic of fear of failure.

Fear of Failure

If you suffer from the fear of failure, you will sabotage yourself in order to not be judged or criticized. If you never hand in your report, you won't get a bad grade. If you never complete the project for your boss, he can't judge it as good or bad. If you never do things that are consistently good for you, you won't feel much better, and you eliminate the risk that it could be taken away from you.

When you suffer from the general fear of failure, typical fears include:

- The fear of making a mistake
- The fear of being judged/criticized
- The fear of being seen as a fraud/imposter
- The fear of being humiliated

Common beliefs include:

- It feels safer to play small
- Failure is inevitable, so why bother

People with the fear of failure are convinced their work will never be perfect enough, so failure is inevitable. It feels safer to play small and stay under the radar because being noticed would inevitably bring criticism and possibly humiliation. Let's tackle some of these fears and beliefs with Tapping.

Tapping Target: Fear of Making a Mistake

If you're afraid of failure, you live in fear of making a mistake, or of someone catching you being imperfect. It's a very stressful way to live. It also keeps you from completing anything at home or at work. As my client said, "I'd rather get an incomplete than a bad grade."

See if you can measure your fear of making a mistake on the 0-10 point scale. You may need to tune in to a past mistake you made that triggered someone's criticism, or the fear of making a mistake in the future. Try this Tapping Sequence:

Side of Hand: Even though I'm afraid of making a mistake, it could be catastrophic, I accept who I am and how I feel. Even though I can't make another mistake, they'll find out I'm a failure, I accept who I am and how I feel about this topic.

Eyebrow: I'm afraid of making a mistake.
Side of Eye: I can't make another mistake.
Under Eye: It would be terrible to make a mistake.
Under Nose: I'd rather not finish the project.
Chin: I'm afraid of making a mistake.
Collarbone: I'd get into trouble.
Under Arm: I don't want to screw up.
Head: I'm afraid of making a mistake.

Take a deep breath, and measure your fear of making a mistake again on the 0-10 point scale. See if any new memories have surfaced, or if the fear has decreased at all and continue Tapping:

Side of Hand: Even though I'm still afraid of making a mistake, I deeply and completely love and accept myself anyway. Even though I'm still afraid of making a mistake, it would feel terrible, I accept who I am and how I feel.

Eyebrow: I'm still afraid I'll make a big mistake.
Side of Eye: I'm still afraid they'll catch my mistakes.
Under Eye: I'm still afraid I'll make another mistake.
Under Nose: I don't want to make a mistake.
Chin: It would be so terrible.
Collarbone: Mistakes are terrible.
Under Arm: I don't want to make another mistake.

Head: I'll do anything to avoid making a mistake.

Take another deep breath, and measure your fear of making a mistake on the 0-10 point scale. Any changes in your feelings? Has the fear decreased at all? You may need to tap on a past mistake that has been lodged in your memory in order to completely neutralize this fear. Your Tapping Target might sound like: "Even though I'm afraid of making another mistake like that one..." Proceed to the Gratitude Tapping below.

Side of Hand: Even though I'm still afraid of making another mistake, I appreciate who I am and how hard I work. Even though I'm still afraid of making another mistake, I appreciate my feelings and how hard I try to do a good job.

Eyebrow: Thank you, Universe, for all the lessons I've learned.
Side of Eye: I'm so grateful for who I am.
Under Eye: Thank you for my knowledge and skills.
Under Nose: Thank you for all my knowledge and skills.
Chin: I appreciate who I am and how I feel.
Collarbone: I'm grateful that nobody is perfect.
Under Arm: Thank you, Universe, for bringing me so much wisdom.
Head: I appreciate all of me, mistakes and all.

Take a final deep breath, and measure your fear of making a mistake on the 0-10 point scale. If this fear hasn't been dramatically decreased, you may need to neutralize a traumatic experience you remember about the consequences of making a mistake in the past. You could start your Tapping with the setup phrase: "Even though I remember how he yelled at me when I made that mistake back then, I deeply and completely love and accept myself anyway..."

Tapping Target: Fear of Being Criticized

The panic some people feel at the thought of making a mistake is followed and made worse by the instantaneous fear of being criticized and judged.

Katie

Katie told me she grew up with two "mean" older brothers. She was constantly criticized by them for everything. She was four years younger than her nearest brother and she said "there was so much room for him to taunt and criticize me." When he was twelve, she was eight, and the gap was perfect for a lonely hurt boy to take his frustrations out on his younger sister. When I asked Katie what her brother would criticize her about, she said "What wouldn't he criticize me about. Everything from my looks to my being alive. He even suggested I was a 'mistake.'"

I taught Katie to use the Tapping for her memories of being hurt, helpless, and criticized. She felt tremendous relief for these old events in her life where she often felt humiliated because her brother would taunt her at school in front of his classmates. Once Katie felt the relief from EFT, she could connect her current sabotage behavior to her fear of being criticized at work. She never spoke up, even when she had good ideas, and was getting increasingly frustrated with not being recognized. Soon the balance between the risk of being criticized and the frustration of holding herself back started to change, and she took remarkable steps forward at work.

The Tapping also made space for Katie to start her gratitude practice. She told me she had never wanted to feel or be grateful about her family, because she thought it would let her brother off the hook for how he had treated her. She was able to forgive him for being immature and hurt, and she blossomed in all her relationships.

Think of a time in your past when you were criticized, and notice if there is any emotional charge connected to it on the 0-10 point scale. If not, imagine being criticized for handing in a future project at work, or for standing out socially, and measure that fear on the 0-10 point scale. Proceed with the Tapping Sequence below:

Side of Hand: Even though I'm afraid of being criticized, I deeply and completely love and accept myself anyway. Even though I'm afraid of being criticized and feeling like a failure, I deeply and completely love and accept myself anyway.

Eyebrow: I'm afraid of being criticized.
Side of Eye: I hate being criticized.
Under Eye: I'm really afraid of being criticized.
Under Nose: I hate being criticized.
Chin: I live in fear of being criticized.
Collarbone: I hate being criticized.
Under Arm: I don't want to be criticized.
Head: I hope I don't get criticized.

Take a deep breath, and measure how afraid of being criticized you are now on the 0-10 point scale. You may need to tune in to a past memory when you felt criticized to measure your fear and distress about it. Do the next round of Tapping:

Side of Hand: Even though I'm still afraid that I might be criticized, no wonder I don't want to start or finish anything, I accept who I am and how I feel. Even though I'm still convinced I'll be criticized, I accept all of my feelings.

Eyebrow: I'm still afraid I'll be criticized again.
Side of Eye: I'm still afraid of being criticized.
Under Eye: I'm so worried I'll be criticized.
Under Nose: I hate being criticized and judged.
Chin: No wonder I get in my own way.
Collarbone: No wonder I won't finish anything.
Under Arm: I'm afraid I'll be criticized again.
Head: I hate being criticized and judged.

Take another deep breath, and measure how afraid you feel about being criticized now on the 0-10 point scale. Proceed to the Gratitude Tapping.

Side of Hand: Even though I get in my own way because I'm afraid I'll be criticized, I accept who I am and how I feel. Even though I'm afraid I'll be criticized and judged, no wonder I keep getting on my own way, I accept who I am and how I feel.

Eyebrow: I'm grateful for how far I've come.
Side of Eye: Thank you, Universe, for so much wisdom along the way.
Under Eye: I appreciate how much I've learned.
Under Nose: Thank you, Universe, for so many opportunities to grow.
Chin: I feel so grateful for these lessons.
Collarbone: I appreciate who I've become.
Under Arm: Thank you, Universe, for all of my life.
Head: I feel grateful for how far I've come.

Take a final deep breath, and measure this fear of being criticized now on the 0-10 point scale. You may continue Tapping on your fear of being criticized, targeting past times you remember as well as your fear of being criticized again in the future.

Tapping Target: Fear of Being Seen as a Fraud

Part of the fear of failure includes imposter syndrome, or the fear of being "found out" as a fraud, that you don't really know enough, and that any success is a fluke. Research shows that up to 82% of people have felt like an imposter in their life.[28] The fear of being found out as an imposter will absolutely shape your thoughts and your behavior.

Measure your fear of "being found out as an imposter/fraud" on the 0-10 point scale. Proceed to the Tapping Round below.

Side of Hand: Even though I'm afraid they'll find out that I don't know what I'm doing, I accept who I am and how I feel. Even though I'm afraid they'll find out that I'm a total imposter, I accept who I am and how I feel.
Eyebrow: I'm afraid they'll figure out that I'm a fraud.
Side of Eye: I'm convinced they'll see right through me.
Under Eye: I'm afraid they'll think I'm an imposter.
Under Nose: I'm afraid they'll think I don't have what it takes.
Chin: I'm convinced they'll see right through me.
Collarbone: What if they see that I'm just a fraud?

Under Arm: I'm afraid they'll think I'm a fraud.
Head: What if they think I'm a fraud?

Take a deep breath, and measure your fear of being "found out" again on the 0-10 point scale. Are there any past events where you felt this strong fear? Tune in to those experiences and measure your fear of that happening *again*.

Side of Hand: Even though I'm still convinced that they'll think I'm just a fraud, I deeply and completely love and accept myself anyway. Even though I'm still convinced that they'll find out I don't know what I'm doing, I accept who I am and how I feel.
Eyebrow: I'm still afraid I'm just an imposter.
Side of Eye: No wonder I'm afraid of failing.
Under Eye: I'm afraid anything I do will fail.
Under Nose: I'm still convinced I'm just a fraud.
Chin: I'm afraid they'll see right through me.
Collarbone: I'm so afraid they'll think I don't know what I'm doing.
Under Arm: I'm still convinced I'll be found out.
Head: No wonder I won't complete anything.

Take another deep breath, and measure your fear of being found out on the 0-10 point scale. It may be helpful to imagine yourself handing in a project to your boss or producing a project that will be seen by others in order to get the accurate rating on the scale. You may keep using Tapping on the above sequences, or proceed to the Gratitude Tapping below.

Side of Hand: Even though I'm still afraid of being seen as an imposter, I choose to remember how far I've come. Even though I'm still afraid of being seen as a fraud, I deeply and completely love and accept myself anyway.
Eyebrow: Thank you for helping me recognize this challenge.
Side of Eye: I'm grateful I've changed so much.
Under Eye: There is so much to be grateful for in my life.
Under Nose: Thank you, Universe, for so much to appreciate.
Chin: Thank you for all the lessons I've learned.
Collarbone: I appreciate who I've become.

Under Arm: I feel grateful for these opportunities.
Head: Thank you, Universe, for so much to appreciate.

Take a final deep breath, and measure your *fear of being found out* on the 0-10 point scale. Continue using Tapping on this fear until it fades so much it no longer bothers you in your professional or personal life.

Tapping Target: I Believe It's Safer to Play Small

If you're afraid of failure, playing small is a solution your unconscious mind will offer you. You won't be seen, judged, or evaluated if no one can see you. When you stay under the radar, there's no risk. Measure how true this belief feels on the 0-10 point scale. You may need to tune in to an old event where you were standing out and you got into "trouble." Proceed to the Tapping Sequences:

Side of Hand: Even though I need to play small so I can be safe, I deeply and completely love and accept myself anyway. Even though I have to play small so I can be safe, I accept who I am and how I feel.

Eyebrow: I want to play small.
Side of Eye: It's smart to play small.
Under Eye: It's safer to play small.
Under Nose: I don't want to be judged.
Chin: It's easier just to play small.
Collarbone: I need to play small.
Under Arm: I want to play small.
Head: Playing small is much safer.

Take a deep breath, and measure how true this belief feels to you now on the 0-10 point scale. If the Tapping Sequences brought up a specific incident where you learned to play small because of the consequences you faced *when you didn't*, use that imagery and memory for the Tapping Rounds.

Side of Hand: Even though it still feels safer playing small, I accept who I am and where I learned this belief. Even though I'm convinced it's safer to play small, I deeply and completely love and accept myself anyway.

Eyebrow: I still need to play small.
Side of Eye: I still know it's safer for me.
Under Eye: Then they can't judge me.
Under Nose: It still feels safer to play small.
Chin: I know it's safer to play small.
Collarbone: I have to play small to be safe.
Under Arm: It's safer to play small.
Head: It's just safer this way.

Take another deep breath, and measure how true this belief feels to you now on the 0-10 point scale. You may also continue Tapping on the memory of the event that taught you it was safer to play small. Proceed to the Gratitude Tapping below.

Side of Hand: Even though I was taught to play small, or I wouldn't be safe, I accept who I am and how I feel. Even though I learned the hard way that it's safer to play small, I accept how I feel and who I am.
Eyebrow: I'm so grateful for the lessons I learned.
Side of Eye: I'm so grateful I can unlearn them now.
Under Eye: I'm grateful I can keep myself safe now.
Under Nose: I love knowing I can keep myself safe.
Chin: I appreciate that I can be safe no matter what.
Collarbone: Thank you, Universe, for keeping me safe now.
Under Arm: Thank you, Universe, for so much healing.
Head: Thank you for all the healing I've done.

Take a final deep breath, and measure how true this belief feels to you now on the 0-10 point scale. You may review these sequences and tap again on whatever memories you have of events where you were taught to play small.

Now we'll move on to the next section and work on blocks that show up as ailments and pain in our physical body.

CHAPTER 8
Health Challenges

Stress, Exhausted Nervous System, Migraine Attacks, Autoimmune Disorders, Fatigue, Insomnia

While physical challenges have not been one of the primary blocks to practicing gratitude for me or my clients over the years, I don't want anything to stand in your way of being able to take advantage of the superpower of gratitude. I think it's worth including a chapter on pain and symptoms, because they also block your ability and desire to reach for healthy habits and practices. If your body is full of aches and pains, it's not natural to reach for healthy habits. If you suffer from an autoimmune disorder, insomnia, or an injury, it's enough to ask yourself to get through the day.

My goal is to offer you another tool to help you with these physical conditions. Over the years, I have witnessed miraculous results in clients' bodies as a result of reducing guilt, resentment, fear, and anger. And while I'm not a doctor, I have also witnessed dramatic reductions in pain and discomfort when clients focus on the emotions and beliefs about their diagnosis, pain, or prognosis. Let's get started.

Tapping Target: Stress and Tension

If you ask someone what stress *feels like* to them, they'll often describe it as tension in some part of their body. They will also describe a kind of monkey mind, or fogginess, where they can't concentrate, feel constantly worried, and aren't very efficient.

How does your stress show up for you? In your body? In your thoughts? In your behavior? Tune in to your body now, and locate where you think you're holding your stress. Now measure how high your discomfort feels on the 0-10 point scale. It doesn't matter whether you call it stress, tension, or agitation, just locate and measure it. Start with this Tapping Round:

Side of Hand: Even though my stress shows up as tension in my body, I deeply and completely love and accept myself anyway. Even though I'm holding all my stress as tension in my body, I accept who I am and how I feel.

Eyebrow: This stress and tension in my body.
Side of Eye: I'm holding the stress as tension in my body.
Under Eye: All this stress and tension in my body.
Under Nose: I feel tight and sore from holding this tension.
Chin: All this stress and tension in my body.
Collarbone: All this stress and tension.
Under Arm: It exhausts me.
Head: My stress shows up as tension in my body.

Take a deep breath, and measure the level of stress and tension now on the 0-10 point scale. Did the sensations change? Did the number go down? At any time, you may substitute your personal description of stress in your own body, for instance: "Even though my stress shows up as tightness in my neck, I deeply and completely love and accept myself anyway."

Side of Hand: Even though I'm still storing all my stress in my body, I accept who I am and how I feel. Even though I'm holding all my stress as tension in my body, I deeply and completely love and accept myself anyway.

Eyebrow: I'm still storing stress in my body.
Side of Eye: I feel so stressed out.
Under Eye: I feel so much tension in my body.
Under Nose: I'm holding so much stress in my body.
Chin: I'm storing stress in my body.
Collarbone: All this stress in my body.
Under Arm: I have way too much stress in my body.
Head: This stress and tension is getting to me.

Take another deep breath, and measure your stress levels again on the 0-10 point scale. You may continue to tap to release the stress and tension you feel in your body, or move on to the Gratitude Tapping.

Side of Hand: Even though I still have all this stress in my body, I accept who I am and how I feel. Even though I still have all this stress and tension in my body, I feel ready to release it now.

Eyebrow: I feel grateful in spite of the stress.
Side of Eye: Thank you, Universe, for my strong body.
Under Eye: I appreciate that I'm releasing the stress now.
Under Nose: Thank you for helping me release my stress.
Chin: Thank you, Universe, for so much to appreciate in my life.
Collarbone: I appreciate my body so much.
Under Arm: I'm grateful for the lessons I've learned.
Head: Thank you, Universe, for showing me what to appreciate.

Take a final deep breath, and measure your stress level now on the 0-10 point scale. I invite you to tap on your stress level for a minimum of 10 minutes a day, including where and how stress shows up in your body.

Lisa

Lisa was a regular talk therapy client of mine. One day she hadn't even reached her chair before she blurted out, "I had a panic attack this morning!" I asked her what her theory was about what had triggered it. She said "Nothing. I'm not anxious, I don't get anxious, and I've never had a panic attack before." Sure enough, she had all the symptoms such as shortness of breath, tightness in her hands and feet, dizziness, and a very dry mouth.

As the conversation continued, Lisa informed me that she had had a huge blowup with her boss. She said she felt enraged and helpless to get him to listen to her concerns. When I asked her if she thought the anger might have triggered her panic attack, she was silent for a moment.

"That's it," she said. "I've never had so much pent up anger in my life. I felt like I was going to explode." Lisa admitted that she hadn't been paying attention to how her stress levels were ramping up, and easily saw how she had reached a tipping point that culminated in a panic attack.

Getting to the trigger for her panic was an excellent first step. Her next steps were to monitor her stress levels, tap on them, identify the signs of her anger bubbling over, and use Tapping and journaling to reduce her rage. Lisa refused to write a gratitude list about her job, but she was able to incorporate gratitude into her life about her relationships, family, and health.

Tapping Target: Exhausted Nervous System

A consequence of prolonged stress is an exhausted nervous system that becomes stretched to its limit. We finally stretch the rubber band so many times that it loses its resiliency and doesn't bounce back. This result can come from living in a stressful environment every day, from having your container too full, or from being hypervigilant, always waiting for something bad to happen. Eventually, our nervous system loses its elasticity and while we also feel wired and agitated, we feel exhausted and spent. Even sleep doesn't restore us.

Even if you don't know or feel as if your nervous system is stretched beyond its limits, I highly recommend trying this Tapping Sequence to speak to your nervous system and give it some relief. In this sequence, we won't measure your before and after feelings on the 0-10 point scale.

Side of Hand: Even though I suspect my nervous system is totally spent, and draining me of all my energy, I deeply and completely love and accept myself. Even though my nervous system is totally spent, I accept who I am and how I feel.

Eyebrow: My nerves are shot.
Side of Eye: I feel exhausted.
Under Eye: I feel wired and tired.
Under Nose: I have no energy.
Chin: I feel anxious all the time.
Collarbone: I'm convinced my nervous system is shot.
Under Arm: I have nothing left.

Head: I feel so spent all the time.

Take a deep breath, and notice how your body feels. Scan your body from your head down to your toes and back again.

Side of Hand: Even though I still feel spent and exhausted, I deeply and completely love and accept myself. Even though I'm totally exhausted and don't know if I can bounce back, I accept who I am and how I feel.

Eyebrow: I know my nerves are spent.
Side of Eye: I feel agitated and exhausted at the same time.
Under Eye: My nerves are spent.
Under Nose: I have nothing left.
Chin: I feel exhausted on a deep level.
Collarbone: My nerves seem shot.
Under Arm: I'm exhausted all the time.
Head: My nerves are shot.

Take another deep breath, and give your body a scan again from the top of your head to the bottom of your feet. There is no right response to this exercise. Just know that you are giving yourself permission to release some of the tension and relax your nerves. Proceed to the Gratitude Tapping below.

Side of Hand: Even though I feel exhausted and spent all the time, I deeply and completely love and accept myself. Even though I feel exhausted and spent most of the time, I choose to appreciate my body now.

Eyebrow: I feel grateful for so much of my life.
Side of Eye: I have so much to appreciate.
Under Eye: I feel exhausted and still feel grateful.
Under Nose: Thank you, Universe, for my strong body.
Chin: Thank you, Universe, for my nervous system.
Collarbone: Thank you, Universe, for showing me my strengths.
Under Arm: I appreciate my health.
Head: Thank you for all my emotions.

Take a final deep breath, and scan your body again. Notice any new sensations or tension leaving your body, and use this Tapping Sequence whenever you feel you are approaching the end of your patience with your nerves.

Pain Relief

Let's say you have a health challenge right now that is stressful, bothersome, and painful, too. You would start with the basics of EFT, and then after you've adequately addressed the target you chose, start expressing statements of gratitude.

When working with health challenges, you can go through any "door" you wish. You may start by using Tapping on the symptom (my throbbing pain), the emotion (I feel hopeless that I'll ever be pain free), the belief (I deserve it), or the behavior (I don't follow doctor's orders).

After Tapping on the basic EFT Round – choosing a target, measuring the distress, using Tapping on the acupoints, re-measuring your distress, doing an additional round – I will offer a round of Gratitude Tapping for you.

Whether you suffer with the symptoms I'm going to address in the Tapping Rounds below or not, I highly recommend you tap along with the scripts for practice, and for the relief you might get for any minor aches and pains. Remember, I am not a doctor, so I'm not treating your diagnosed disease. I'm treating the underlying emotions, beliefs, and behaviors that contribute to your discomfort.

Migraine Attacks

Let's say you're one of the 37 million people in the US that live with the debilitating health challenge of migraine attacks. (American Migraine Foundation).[29] The most common complaints are: a severe throbbing headache, sensitivity to noise and light, and nausea. Living with this syndrome is incredibly challenging, and when a migraine hits, it's very limiting to your life.

Angel

Angel worked in my office building. I noticed he was squinting and seemed uncomfortable. When I asked him what was going on, he said: "I'm having one of my intense headaches again." Apparently, Angel had these several times a week, and they were often 9 or 10 on the intensity scale. The other building workers knew about them because he regularly had to take unscheduled breaks and go lie down on the workmen's couch during the day. I was brand new to Tapping and was eager to try it out on him. During his next break, he came up to my office and I taught him how to use Tapping. He squirmed around when I told him to repeat after me, "I deeply and completely love and accept myself" but I asked him just to repeat the words and tap on his points. After just a few minutes of Tapping, his pain had been reduced dramatically.

When I followed up with him the next week, and weeks and months later, he reported that he never had a 9 or 10 headache again! He said, "I don't know what you did but it worked." While I probably shouldn't have worked on a handyman in my building on his break without all the necessary introductions and practice parameters, I took the risk and it paid off. I will never forget the surprise and delight on his face. He was my first migraine case, but definitely far from my last!

Let's address the throbbing headache pain in this next Tapping Round. You can either wait until you feel a migraine coming on, or tap while you tune in to the experience of the last one you experienced. Measure the level of pain on the 0-10 point scale, and start your Tapping.

Side of Hand: Even though I have this throbbing headache right now, I deeply and completely love and accept myself anyway. Even though I'm struggling with this throbbing headache, I accept who I am and how I feel.

Eyebrow: I have this throbbing headache pain.
Side of Eye: This throbbing headache pain.
Under Eye: My head is pounding.
Under Nose: I can feel it getting worse.
Chin: I know I have a migraine coming on.

Collarbone: I hate this feeling.
Under Arm: I can't stand the pain.
Head: I have this throbbing migraine.

Take a deep breath, and measure how bad the pain is now on the 0-10 point scale. Did it increase? Decrease? Or stay the same? Continue with the Tapping:

Side of Hand: Even though I still have this throbbing headache right now, I deeply and completely accept my body and myself. Even though I'm still struggling with this painful headache, I accept who I am and how I feel.
Eyebrow: I still have this throbbing pain.
Side of Eye: This throbbing headache pain.
Under Eye: My head is pounding.
Under Nose: This pounding headache.
Chin: I know this migraine pain.
Collarbone: This pounding migraine.
Under Arm: This throbbing pain.
Head: This throbbing migraine.

Take a deep breath, and measure the pain again on the 0-10 point scale. Notice if there have been any changes in the level of pain or the location of the symptoms. You may continue with several more rounds of this Tapping or proceed to the Gratitude Tapping Sequence below.

Side of Hand: Even though I have this throbbing migraine pain, I accept who I am and how I feel. Even though I can feel this painful headache coming on, I accept who I am and how I feel.
Eyebrow: I appreciate my body even with this pain.
Side of Eye: Thank you, Universe, for so much to appreciate.
Under Eye: I appreciate my general good health.
Under Nose: Thank you, Universe, for my strong body.
Chin: Thank you, Universe, for the relief that I feel.
Collarbone: I'm grateful for my general health.
Under Arm: Thank you for showing me what to appreciate.

Head: I appreciate how I handle these headaches.

Take another deep breath, measure the migraine pain on the 0-10 point scale, and keep using Tapping on any other symptoms or sensations you are experiencing. I highly recommend you reach for your Tapping points whenever you get the first hint of a migraine. Now let's move on to an emotion you might have about struggling with the pain.

Tapping Target: Pain and Helplessness

Now let's address the emotion you feel when you have pain of any kind. Whether you've had an injury, or you have an illness that produces pain, how do you feel? Hopeless? Helpless? Angry? Anxious? I've heard all of these responses from my clients. We'll address the feeling of helplessness in this next Tapping Sequence.

First, measure how helpless you feel when the pain starts. If you suffer from chronic pain, see if you can measure how helpless you feel about your general pain on the 0-10 point scale. Start the Tapping Round below:

Side of Hand: Even though I feel totally helpless about the pain I feel in my body, I accept who I am and how I feel. Even though I feel totally helpless that I'll ever be pain free in my life, I accept who I am and how I feel.
Eyebrow: I feel so helpless about this pain.
Side of Eye: I feel so helpless about my bodily pain.
Under Eye: Once it starts, I can't do anything.
Under Nose: I feel so helpless about this pain.
Chin: I feel helpless and alone.
Collarbone: I feel helpless and out of control.
Under Arm: I feel so helpless about the pain.
Head: I'm tired of feeling helpless.

Take a deep breath, and measure how helpless you feel about the physical pain now on the 0-10 point scale. Is it still as high as it was before? Continue with the Tapping:

Side of Hand: Even though I feel totally helpless about my physical pain, I accept who I am and how I feel. Even though I feel totally helpless about changing this pain, I accept who I am and how I feel.

Eyebrow: I still feel so helpless about my pain.
Side of Eye: I still feel so helpless about the pain.
Under Eye: Once it starts, I can't do anything.
Under Nose: I still feel helpless about my health.
Chin: I still feel helpless and frustrated.
Collarbone: I feel helpless about the pain.
Under Arm: I feel so helpless once it starts.
Head: I'm tired of feeling helpless.

Take a deep breath and measure your feeling of helplessness again on the 0-10 point scale. Now proceed to the Gratitude Tapping Sequence below.

Side of Hand: Even though I feel helpless over my physical pain, I want to remember how grateful I feel about my general health. Even though I feel helpless once the pain starts, I have decided to remember how grateful I feel about my strength and health.

Eyebrow: I feel grateful for my general health.
Side of Eye: Thank you, Universe, for my strong body.
Under Eye: I appreciate how I handle my pain symptoms.
Under Nose: Thank you, Universe, for advancements in treatment.
Chin: I appreciate who I am even though I'm in pain.
Collarbone: Thank you, Universe, for my general good health.
Under Arm: I love feeling grateful about my body.
Head: Thank you, Universe, for so much to appreciate.

Take a final deep breath, and measure how helpless you feel now on the 0-10 point scale, and continue using Tapping when necessary. In addition, go back and measure your physical pain again and see where it lands now on the 0-10 point scale. You may continue to work with the emotions around your pain or tap on the symptom itself. Be specific: "My stabbing pain," or "My shooting pain in my knee" etc.

Autoimmune Disorders

Let's move on to another health challenge. I found an astounding statistic: 1 in 15 people in the US suffer from an autoimmune disorder.[30] The Cleveland Clinic has identified over 100 autoimmune disorders.[31] If you are suffering with an autoimmune disorder, your immune system attacks your own body, rather than defending against outside intruders such as germs and bacteria. Your immune system becomes both overactive and misdirected.

The most common autoimmune disorders you have likely heard of or suffer from include:

Lupus
Multiple Sclerosis
Rheumatoid Arthritis
Psoriasis
Type 1 diabetes
Irritable Bowel Syndrome
Celiac disease
Graves' disease

There are many "common" symptoms of an autoimmune disorder. They can affect your nervous system, your skin, your endocrine system, your joints, or your muscles. Some of the most common symptoms are fatigue, inflammation, pain, and soreness.

Tapping Target: Fatigue

I'm going to lead you through EFT Tapping Rounds about the common symptom of fatigue that accompanies most autoimmune disorders, followed by a Gratitude Tapping Round.

First, measure how fatigued you feel right now on the 0-10 point scale. If people with a lot of energy would measure 0, where are you?

Side of the hand: Even though my disorder is causing all this fatigue, and I'm so tired of it, I accept who I am and how I feel. Even though I can't stand this relentless fatigue, I accept who I am and how I feel anyway.

Eyebrow: I feel deep fatigue.
Side of Eye: I'm so tired.
Under Eye: I can barely move.
Under Nose: My fatigue feels so deep.
Chin: I feel so tired.
Collarbone: I feel exhausted all the time.
Under Arm: Sleep doesn't seem to help.
Head: I'm tired all the time.

Take a deep breath, and measure your level of fatigue again. Notice if there have been any changes in the sensations or impressions of fatigue. Notice if you feel any energy moving through your body, or any sensations of warmth or coolness.

Side of the hand: Even though I still feel this deep fatigue, and I'm so tired of it, I accept who I am anyway. Even though I suffer from this relentless fatigue, I accept who I am and how I feel.

Eyebrow: I feel deeply fatigued all the time.
Side of Eye: I'm so tired all the time.
Under Eye: I feel such fatigue.
Under Nose: It never seems to stop.
Chin: I feel so tired all the time.
Collarbone: I feel exhausted every day.
Under Arm: No matter what I do I feel tired.
Head: I'm tired all the time.

Take another deep breath, and see if you can measure this symptom of fatigue in your body on the 0-10 point scale, and then proceed to the Gratitude Tapping below.

Side of the hand: Even though I feel this deep fatigue, I also feel grateful for my body and my life. Even though I suffer from this relentless fatigue, I also feel grateful of so much goodness in my life.

Eyebrow: I still feel grateful about my body.

Side of Eye: I don't have to ignore my gratitude.

Under Eye: I feel such gratitude in spite of the fatigue.

Under Nose: Thank you, Universe, for so much gratitude in my life.

Chin: Thank you, Universe, for so much to appreciate in my life.

Collarbone: Thank you for so much gratitude in my life.

Under Arm: I love feeling grateful.

Head: I appreciate so much about my life.

Take a final deep breath, and measure your fatigue now on the 0-10 point scale. You may go back to these Tapping Sequences any time and replace one symptom for another, or add an emotion, belief, or behavior you need to tap on to get relief.

Tapping Target: Insomnia

Insomnia was the first health challenge I cleared with Tapping. I was new to EFT and offered it to my clients who came in with high anxiety, stress, and cravings. I taught my clients how to use it for their symptoms and emotions, and I ended up experiencing surprising benefits as well. While I didn't target my own insomnia or the feelings and conflicts that kept me up at night, I had calmed down my nervous system enough by modeling and leading clients through the Tapping Rounds that it calmed down my anxiety and my nervous system, and my insomnia disappeared.

If you suffer from insomnia, you might want to answer these questions first so you know what to tap on. Using the target phrase "Even though I suffer from insomnia..." isn't targeted enough. You need to identify the feelings, conflicts, or traumas that keep you up at night.

- What work anxiety keeps you awake at night?
- What are you afraid of if you sleep deeply?
- What family concerns keep you up at night?

- What unresolved feelings (anger, guilt, worry) keep you up at night?

For this exercise, we'll use the term anxiety, but for subsequent rounds of Tapping, you can go back and insert your own feelings or conflicts that surfaced when you answered the questions. If you're about to go to bed now, go ahead and use this round for your anxiety from the day that may be lingering in your mind and keeping you awake. You may also use your anxiety about not being able to fall asleep as a target. Go ahead and measure that concern on the 0-10 point scale.

Side of Hand: Even though my anxiety keeps me up at night, I don't feel calm enough to fall asleep, I deeply and completely love and accept myself anyway. Even though I feel so anxious at night because I can't fall asleep, I accept all my feelings anyway.

Eyebrow: I feel so anxious at night.
Side of Eye: Then I feel anxious about not sleeping.
Under Eye: I really need to fall asleep.
Under Nose: I feel so anxious when I go to bed.
Chin: I feel restless and unable to fall asleep.
Collarbone: I feel so anxious when it's time for bed.
Under Arm: I don't want to let go.
Head: I feel so anxious about falling asleep.

Take a deep breath, and measure the level of anxiety you feel now on the 0-10 point scale about having trouble sleeping at night. Continue your Tapping:

Side of Hand: Even though I feel so anxious at night that I can't fall asleep, I deeply and completely love and accept myself anyway. Even though I feel so anxious about not being able to fall asleep, I accept who I am and how I feel.

Eyebrow: I feel so anxious at night.
Side of Eye: I'm so worried about everything.
Under Eye: I can't fall asleep at night.

Under Nose: I hate it when I can't fall asleep.
Chin: I feel so agitated at night.
Collarbone: I'm worried about my insomnia.
Under Arm: I'm worried about my anxiety.
Head: I'm worried I'll never be able to sleep deeply.

Take another deep breath, and measure your anxiety about not being able to fall asleep on the 0-10 point scale. If another target surfaces such as a fight in your family, a resentment towards a friend or colleague, or a feeling of anxiety about an event in the future, go ahead and reword the target to fit your situation. Proceed to the Gratitude Tapping below.

Side of Hand: Even though I'm so anxious about my insomnia, I deeply and completely love and accept myself anyway. Even though I feel so anxious about my insomnia, I accept who I am and how I feel.
Eyebrow: I feel so grateful even though I have insomnia.
Side of Eye: I feel so grateful about so much in my life.
Under Eye: Thank you, Universe, for so much to appreciate.
Under Nose: I appreciate that I'm letting go more.
Chin: I'm grateful that I'm letting go of my worries.
Collarbone: I appreciate how much sleep I do get.
Under Arm: Thank you, Universe, for all that I have in my life.
Head: Thank you, Universe, for the sleep I do get.

Take a final deep breath and measure your concern about your insomnia on the 0-10 point scale. If any other specific concerns came up that you know keep your mind racing at night, go ahead and formulate new target statements and Tapping Rounds for them as well.

In this chapter, we tackled stress, an overloaded nervous system, migraine pain, helplessness about pain, body fatigue, and insomnia. You may substitute any of your health challenges, symptoms, or emotions about your condition, your diagnosis, and your prognosis, for what I've written for you here.

Now let's move on to Part 4 where I'll introduce you to 5 special guests with amazing gratitude stories, and give you my top 7 gratitude exercises that will help you enhance every part of your life.

PART FOUR
STORIES AND INVITATIONS

CHAPTER 9
Before and After Stories

Many thanks to these following contributors who shared their **Before and After Stories** showcasing their experiences of using gratitude in their life. I feel honored that these colleagues and friends agreed to contribute their stories to *Yes, Thank You.*

Sara Connell

The writer Ann Lamott says there are only three prayers: "Help!" "Wow!" and "Thank You!"

Until my late twenties, I sporadically offered these three in what are called "foxhole" prayers. When something big or wonderful or terrible or challenging would arise, I'd yelp my *help wow thank-yous* to whatever I thought was listening and hope for the best.

When I finally decided to address my significant childhood trauma, one of the practices my therapist recommended (as did every one of the self-help books I had begun consuming like a tornado) was a daily gratitude practice. I was up for anything that could lift me out of the tangle of despair and paralysis that the rape, assaults and general dysfunction of my first 18 years had left me in, so I began writing a list of five things every night for which I was grateful. I liked this practice so much I began doing a gratitude list at the start of my morning journaling (another practice I'd adopted per the therapy, 12 step, self-help, spirituality retreats) that had now become my lifestyle. After even 30 days, there was no doubt in my mind that directing my brain away from worry, stress, fear, anxiety, and emotional pain was good for me, and was helping me transform.

My life in all areas improved. I got married, published my first book, moved to London - a lifelong dream! I used gratitude to fall asleep, counting "gratitudes." After years of insomnia, I was falling asleep easily and quickly most nights.

Then, in 2007, after doing 2 years of fertility treatments, I got pregnant with twin boys! It was easy to make my daily gratitude lists during those first two trimesters: tiny, powerful heartbeats, an ultrasound where one of our boys was sucking his thumb! Picking out strollers, matching bassinets, baby sneakers. As we crossed into trimester three, I went into premature labor and the babies came early, stillborn. During the C-section there were complications. I woke up with my children dead and my uterus and bowel cut through. I lost so much blood I needed transfusions. When I got home and was able to move around again, we dismantled the nursery and donated the double sets of onesies and soft blue blankets. Every time the phone rang, I braced my body while another friend shared that she was pregnant. Making a gratitude list felt hard.

I knew the only way through this time was in continuing my spiritual practices. I heard about a technique called "exaggerated gratitude." You take the simplest things- not the big things - and focus all your attention on what you love about them. Drinking a hot cup of tea for example becomes: "I am SOOOOOOOO grateful for this tea. It's so warm. It's so spicy and delicious." The sunlight falling on my face. The dumb Will Farrell movie that made me laugh after I'd cried for three hours on the floor, getting my stitches out and being able to work out again. The point was to go over the top with "I'M SOOOOOO GRATEFUL" and the wild thing was, I started to feel better. The fist of my heart softened for a few minutes after each round of this over the top gratitude. There is no doubt this practice accelerated my recovery and opened me to the miracles to come. The birth of my son, building a company I love and believe in to multi 7 figures a year, leading transformational writing retreats all over the world, being a channel for real, positive impact on our clients' lives.

Twenty-five years after making that first gratitude list, I still start my day with gratitude. My evening practice has evolved into what I call a "win streak" inspired by the author Dan Sullivan. Each evening I give thanks for the biggest "wins" of the day. Then I give "future gratitude" for the intentions I set for the coming 24 hours. I heard a doctor say once that "gratitude is a causative energy." It lowers our blood pressure, improves relationships, increases financial abundance, even helps us live longer. "It's science," he said. To me, it's just magic.

Sara Connell, 5x Best-Selling Author, Founder of Thought Leader Academy

Advait Shah

Gratitude has become an integral part of my daily practice. I was introduced to it by my Reiki teacher, who advised me to actively cultivate gratitude rather than practice it occasionally. One of the most profound ways I use gratitude is by thanking the people who have inspired me, even if I may never be able to reach out to them. Sometimes, I write emails expressing my gratitude, even if they remain in my drafts. The act itself is powerful—it acknowledges the impact they've had on my journey.

But gratitude isn't just limited to people. I also practice gratitude for non-living things that have supported me in ways I once overlooked. For instance, my car has been with me for nine years. It has given me shelter, protection during unpredictable weather, and the freedom to move toward new opportunities. I am deeply grateful for it, for its makers, and for every person who has worked on its maintenance.

Gratitude has transformed my perspective. It helped me shift from focusing on what was missing in my life to appreciating what was already present. I used to stumble upon different things without any real passion, feeling unsure about my path. But gratitude led me to something meaningful—my talk show, *Extreme Gratitude*.

I have always loved talking to people from different domains, and one night, the idea struck me—why not start a podcast dedicated to gratitude? What started as a simple thought turned into a passion project that gave me a purpose. Through my interviews, I get to amplify the voices of those who have turned their struggles into strength. Every shared story reaffirms my belief that gratitude is not just a practice—it's a power that transforms lives.

Before practicing gratitude, I was lost, unsure of my purpose, and burdened with self-doubt and unforgiveness—both toward myself and others. Now that I practice gratitude, my life is full of purpose, fulfillment, and deep appreciation for the journey.

Whenever I get overwhelmed or stressed out, I use *Emotional Freedom Techniques* (EFT) as a tool to calm down my thoughts and simply say the words "Thank you" on all the Tapping points. When you use EFT while practicing gratitude, your conscious mind is fully aware of what you are doing, making the practice even more effective. This combination has helped me deepen my gratitude practice, bringing clarity and peace into my life.

I have come to understand that prayer should not just be about asking; it should be about thanking—thanking God for what He has given, what He is giving, and what He will give.

If you haven't already, I urge you to practice gratitude. It can move mountains. It can bring hope when everything seems uncertain. And most importantly, it can open doors you never even knew existed. That's why I named my podcast *Extreme Gratitude*—because gratitude is not just a feeling; it's a way of life.

Advait Shah, Founder, Extreme Gratitude Podcast

Christina Nylese

Prior to getting sober in 2011, after a good ten years of destructive drinking and losing everything I worked for, I never gave gratitude a second thought. Of course, I told my parents "thank you" when I got a generous check in my Christmas stocking every year. I said "thank you" when given a compliment. I recited my prayers every night and told God, "Thank you for everything you've given me." But it was all just words. There was never a felt experience of gratitude, and I hadn't yet learned how powerful that could be and how it would play a critical role in my transformation one day.

I was given everything I needed and more growing up. I didn't know what it was like to live without things, except for the time when my parents wouldn't buy me an Atari, or a Cabbage Patch Kid, when all of my friends at school had them. In an attempt to not spoil me too much, they put me on their own "waiting list" just to remind me that money didn't grow on trees. But I still thought it did. I spent my summers in our oceanfront beach house, I went on at least one vacation a year, always staying in five-star resorts, and ate at some of the finest New York City restaurants at a very early age. Dad paid for college and graduate school, leaving me debt free as I entered adulthood. My dad liked to spend money on material things, and he liked letting you know it. The showiness started to bother me, and feeling gratitude for material things felt icky or wrong. Although I had no complaints about my way of life, I didn't need material things to be happy, but apparently he did.

The first time I can remember feeling true gratitude was when I found myself standing in a homeless shelter, believe it or not. I was only a few days sober, fresh out of detox, with no place to live. This was far from living modestly, and I had to start over that day with only seven dollars in my pocket, just enough for a bed for the week. I was at such a low point in my life. I had nothing left, yet I felt happier than I had in a long time. How could that be?

Alcoholism took everything from me. I lived like I was a victim for years, mad at the world for doing me wrong. "Why me?" I'd ask. During those years I took from everyone, never showing appreciation for anything. Even in my darkest days drunk, I didn't know what it felt like to be without what I needed. I didn't know what it felt like to not have love and support and compassion. I lived knowing my parents would always pick up my messy pieces. They had always given me what I needed. But not this time.

And thank goodness! To this day, I hold so much gratitude in my heart for the "abandonment" I felt that day. It saved my life. When I found myself with so little to survive on, I discovered the true essence of gratitude. It was so easy to be grateful for the little things - the coffee in the morning, a bed to sleep in, a bike to ride so I could get to where I needed to go. I'd get up at sunrise and enjoy the peace of the morning with a journal. I'd relish time on the beach just a few miles down the road. I felt appreciation for the new friends I was making in my recovery meetings.

Growing up with somewhat of a silver spoon in my mouth didn't make adjusting to homelessness easy. But without this experience, I wouldn't have discovered the felt experience of gratitude. It was a different kind of feeling, all tied up with hope and excitement for what was yet to come. I truly believe that connecting with gratitude during those first few days at the homeless shelter gave me the power to be resilient, to thrive, and to live with appreciation for all of God's gifts, big and small.

Christina Nylese, Holistic Health and Recovery Coach
Best-Selling Author, *Self-Love, Self-Healing*

Debbie Forcier-Lynn

You are always Expanding. WHAT are you expanding?

Gratitude IS my connection to manifesting the life I desire. What do I WANT to expand? I do this through my "Get To Grateful" practice. This practice isn't just about making an "I am grateful for" list. It's about shifting my belief the moment I realize I am off and not expanding what I want. When you get to the space of grateful, no matter WHAT the situation, you arrive at the space of solutions, intentional expansion, opportunity, and possibility. It moves you directly into wisdom and creation.

I like to think of gratitude as the fairy dust of appreciation. I didn't realize there was a difference between gratitude and appreciation until my eternal friend, Tricia invited me to a new thought. When I sprinkle gratitude on my thoughts, actions, and emotions, I am able to stand in awe and appreciation for my experience, and all judgment fades. Even in gratitude, there is a glimpse of judgment because we are "looking for the grateful." Once you cross the grateful bridge and it sprinkles its magic, you ARE! You no longer have to look for the grateful because it is the IS.

Here's how it works for me: If I experience something that triggers a thought, emotion, or action I do not want, my first response is, *"Get to Grateful, Debbie."* Sometimes, this shift happens instantly, a quick mental reframe that gets me back on track. But more often than not, I have to grab my journal and get the experience up and out on paper. This first pass? It's not pretty. It's my "verbal rant," just dumping everything out, raw and unfiltered. Giving yourself a time limit is usually best so as not to wallow and give it any more power.

Once all the junk is out, I take a breath, close my eyes, and ask myself:

- "WHAT do you WANT?" What will make you feel your BEST, your HIGHEST?

I sit with that. I hold the vision. And when I get clarity, I write it down. Then I ask:

- "Teach me" or as another friend taught me, "show me" how to align with THAT energy from where I am right now?"

I listen. I find the next step. And then I take it.

Finally, I write my "Get to Grateful" statement. And here's the best part: I do it because I am GREAT-FULL. When you are FULL of GREAT, guess what? YOU and everything around you is GREAT.

This practice has changed everything for me. It keeps me in a place of empowered, intentional expansion. When I DON'T do it, I can feel myself slipping into doubt, stuck in problems, caught in lack, and weighed down by limitations. Staying committed to the practice, I stay in flow, in creation, and in alignment with the life I desire to live.

Gratitude isn't just a feel-good exercise; it's a transformational practice, habit, and way of BEing and DOing. It is no longer a thought; it is as connected to me as my right arm. I don't choose in the morning whether I'll go out with my arm today or leave it on the nightstand.

There is no other option or choice. I AM this practice; this is my BE, DO, HAVE practice of living. In the beginning, it took focus and conscious choice, and as I was faithful to my commitment, it completely rewired how I saw and SEE challenges as opportunities. It's the fuel that keeps my expansion on track and helps me show up for my life, work, and the people around me with intention, focus, and purpose.

So here's my challenge to you: Get to Grateful. What are you expanding today? Choose to expand appreciation, solutions, and possibilities. When you do, you'll find that life responds in kind, because when you're **Great-Full**, you're **FULL of GREAT, and great things happen.**

Debbie Forcier-Lynn, CEO, Cultural Alignment Solutions

Amanda Hinman

At the age of thirty-three, I was perpetually exhausted and anxious. My hair was thinning, acne peppered my chin, and mood swings were a daily occurrence, yet I thought these symptoms could all be explained by my fourth pregnancy in six years.

I sat up with a bolt of defiance when the doctor diagnosed me with an autoimmune disease called Hashimoto's Thyroiditis and explained that my poor thyroid health could be detrimental to the growing baby. This news was a total shock because I had always considered myself very healthy. I ate salads five days a week, didn't consume meat very often, and was a group fitness instructor. How could this be happening?

The standard of care for thyroid disease at that time was to take medication for life. My doctor explained that this condition was hereditary and the likelihood of additional autoimmune diseases in future years was significantly higher.

The emotions of defeat and anger became regular visitors in my life. I believed my body had betrayed me and was attacking itself. I spewed things like "STOP crying and calm down" to my 6-year-old daughter when she couldn't tie her shoe. Of course, my behavior was not modeling calm presence, yet I expected her to learn what that was…go figure.

Twenty months later, I found myself completely hopeless, gripping the plastic visitor's chair with my stone-cold fingers in a hospital room, listening to a pediatric neurologist explain that my daughter needed to take anti-seizure medication for life. This was in the aftermath of her fourth seizure in the past 12 hours. I didn't understand what had happened to my seemingly healthy daughter. She had always been sensitive and struggled with anxiety, but nothing debilitating yet. I was terrified.

Something deep inside of me knew there was more to the story of why I developed an auto-immune condition, and she had developed seizures. There had to be root causes I was missing. This path inadvertently led to one of the greatest gifts in my life. The gift of gratitude.

I went back to school to study functional medicine science to learn how to help my daughter and me. Functional medicine is an individualized, patient-centric, science-based approach to healthcare that looks beyond symptom resolution to identify why illness occurs, address those root causes, and restore health.

Studying the interconnectedness of the body's various systems was awe-inspiring. I shifted from experiencing daily defeat and anger to feeling curious to learn more about the immense complexity, organization, and intelligence of the human body. It was truly remarkable.

I appreciated a new understanding of how my daughter's body and my body had not been getting enough valuable nutrients to synthesize neurotransmitters and detoxify stress hormones. Learning which factors in our lifestyle had created imbalances in our bodies became liberating.

I appreciated that previously, many aspects of our health were not optimal. I felt empowered to positively impact the areas that we had unintentionally neglected. Each day, I wrote in my journal three things that I valued about my physical or emotional health.

"Thank you taste buds for allowing me to enjoy my sweet potato, spinach and scrambled egg skillet!" "I love how my legs are sore from the leg squats and lunges yesterday…they are getting stronger." "I appreciated the sense of stillness and mental ease during my meditation tonight." "It's fun to see how my daughter cried out her worry this afternoon. Her body is intelligent and lets the stress flow out of her." These are examples of the gratitude I documented and captured in my yellow daily journal.

Increasing awareness and focusing on the positive aspects of our health created a ripple effect. Weeks folded into months of giving grateful acknowledgement to our bodies, and we began to heal. Within 9 months we had rebuilt our health through the combination of customized nutritional improvements, adjustments to stress management habits and daily gratitude which expanded our appreciation of health. Both my daughter, and I weaned off all medications and have maintained vibrant health for the past 10 years.

I believe gratitude comes from first, increasing familiarity with an area you desire change, and second, building consistent acknowledgement of the real time experience of that area of your life. In my health journey this looked like learning more about the miraculous design of the human body through studying functional medicine science and then daily acknowledgement of the real time experience of the body in action.

Gratitude played a significant role in my family's health transformation and has been contagious! Now, I eagerly look for other areas in my life where I can increase my understanding and acknowledgement to enjoy even more fulfillment.

Amanda Hinman, AFMC, Women's Hormone Health Expert & Coach
Best-Selling Author, *The Thyroid and Hormone Solution*

CHAPTER 10
Gratitude Invitations

All in all, science confirms that the life-giving practice of gratitude broadens our lives by enabling healing of the past, providing contentment in the present, and delivering hope for the future.

Robert A. Emmons, *Gratitude Works!*[32]

There are dozens of ways to express your gratitude – through writing, out loud, with a friend, or during a meditation. Over the years, I have compiled my list of favorites, and narrowed it down to my top 7 ways to express gratitude. I have described them for you in this chapter.

#1 - Daily Gratitude Journaling

This is probably the most common and most recommended form of expressing gratitude. This is a freeform style of journaling for between 3-10 minutes every day about what you feel grateful for and what you appreciate in your life. You may write paragraphs, sentences, bullet points, or even a story about how yesterday or today unfolded for you. Notice the feelings in your body as you express your gratitude. Honor this practice by getting yourself a special pen and a unique notebook, and carving out private time to do this journaling.

#2 - Gratitude List

I've done this practice for years, and have notebooks filled with gratitude lists. All I do is number 1-10, and list every item, experience, or person I feel grateful for today. It doesn't matter if your list doesn't change from day to day. I recommend focusing on smaller items as well. For example, not just appreciating a roof over my head, which is amazing, but items such as "I'm so grateful I had enough time to get the laundry done before my meeting."

My other favorite variations of this list include:
- 10 things I love about my life
- 10 things I appreciate about my life
- 10 things I appreciate about myself
- 10 things that make me feel relief right now

Counting your blessings is another variation on the theme of making a gratitude list, and any time we add a twist, it invites something different to come forward from our mind and focus. Write out what you consider to be the top blessings in your life. They can be from your past or your current life. You could say "I feel blessed by the way I was raised by my parents," or "It's such a blessing that I landed in a profession that I love," or "My dog was such a blessing for me when I was sick."

Popular phrases I use are: "Thank you for all the blessings I have in my life and all the blessings I am receiving" and "I am blessed with unlimited abundance."

And Bob Proctor taught his followers to say: "I am so happy and grateful now that…" and fill in the blanks after that.

#3 - Gratitude Interview

I love this gratitude practice. Ask a friend or colleague to conduct a mock interview with you. You may write out the questions ahead of time, or let them wing it. Here are some examples of the questions:

- Tell me why gratitude is important to you.
- What are the top 3 things you feel grateful for in your life?
- What are the top 3 aspects of your career that you appreciate?
- Who are the top 3 people you feel grateful for in your life?
- What aspects of your health do you appreciate most?

- What aspects of your job do you appreciate most?
- What are the top 3 features of your home that you appreciate?

#4 - Guess What? Letter

This letter could be written to yourself, to a friend, or a colleague. The beauty of this practice is that we're writing as if what we want has already come to pass. Studies have shown that our body doesn't know the difference between an imagined and a real event. This means that writing this letter can produce the same chemicals and positive feelings as if the success already happened. (I first published this gratitude practice in my book, *Attracting Abundance with EFT*.)

- Guess what? I'm so grateful that I was able to publish my book and become a best-selling author!
- Guess what? I'm so grateful that I was able to lose the last 10 pounds.
- Guess what? I'm so busy in my coaching practice I had to start a waiting list.
- Guess what? I'm so grateful that I resolved that conflict with my friend.
- Guess what? I'm so grateful that I finally sold my house to the perfect family.

#5 - Gratitude - Out Loud

I use this version of a gratitude practice on my morning speed walks. It's as simple as it sounds. While I'm walking around the park in New York, I notice nature, other people, quirky New York scenes, and talk out loud about my gratitude. It might sound like this:

I'm so grateful for all the beautiful trees in the park.

I'm so grateful that I get to see these adorable dogs playing in the park.

I'm so grateful the daffodils are starting to come up.

I'm so grateful it's not that crowded at this time of day.

#6 - Gratitude Meditation

I confess to having a difficult time staying present during my morning meditations. I often turn the time into a Gratitude Meditation. All I do is set my timer, close my eyes, and recite my "gratitudes" for my life. You may use background music if you prefer, but notice how you feel in your body and your mind as your expressions of gratitude keep flowing through you.

#7 - Gratitude Gridwork

I learned the term "gridwork" from the creators of the Abraham-Hicks website, Esther and Jerry Hicks. Esther Hicks is a channeler, and until his passing, her husband Jerry Hicks was the one who asked the questions for her and her guides to answer. Esther now offers weekly YouTube videos and live workshops around the world. After a few months of teaching what I thought was their exercise called gridwork, I discovered that I had misinterpreted what they were asking their audiences to do. No harm done, it's close. And I teach this technique in all my live workshops around the world.

Take a piece of paper and draw a huge square on it, reaching to the top, bottom, and both sides. Inside this large square, draw 3 equidistant horizontal lines. Then draw 3 equidistant vertical lines. You should now have a grid of 16 boxes, 4 across and 4 up and down. See image below.

Gratitude Grid

In these boxes, write words, experiences, or feelings that you would really appreciate noticing today. Sometimes I write at the top of the box, *Things I'd love to feel today.*

For instance: I often write *happiness* in one of the boxes...*relief* in another...*humor* in another...*lightness* in another. By the end you will have filled in all 16 boxes with wonderful feelings that you want to experience in your life today.

You may also write an aspect of your life at the top, so that if your focus is on your job today, you would fill in the 16 boxes around your work life. Or focus on your relationship and ask yourself: *what would I like to feel about my relationship today*...and fill in the boxes.

Those are my top 7 gratitude practices. I highly recommend doing at least one a day. You may also, of course, incorporate your Gratitude Lists while you're Tapping, a form of habit stacking.

Now let's proceed to the 30-Day Gratitude Challenge. I hope you'll join me. You may start any day you wish, and try to keep it going for 30 days.

Please scan this QR code or visit your *Yes, Thank You* book portal at www.theyescode.com/thankyou for supporting materials for this book.

PART FIVE
THE CHALLENGE

CHAPTER 11

30-Day Gratitude Challenge

*Acknowledging the good that is already
in your life is the foundation for all abundance.*

Eckhart Tolle, Author: A New Earth [33]

Welcome to your **30-Day Gratitude Challenge**. This is an incredible opportunity to improve your daily life. It's harder than you think to stick to new habits every day; that's why I call this a *challenge*. But the benefits will be overwhelmingly positive if you can stick with it...they have been for me.

How to Use This 30-Day Gratitude Challenge

I have organized this special section for you to make this challenge as easy as possible.

During the first 14 days of Week 1 and 2, I invite you to follow along with the exercises I have provided – you can see it as a restaurant menu – with an appetizer, a main course, and of course, dessert.

Your Appetizer

- Fill out your Gratitude Grid (see directions in this chapter).

Your Main Course

- Complete your daily Tapping Sequences, including Gratitude or Thank You Tapping.
- I have provided full Tapping Sequences for Days 1-14.
- From Day 15-30, choose whichever Tapping Target you prefer from either Days 1-14, Chapters 5-8, or make up one of your own.

Your Dessert
- Write a Gratitude List.
- Choose one of the specific lists I have provided for Days 1-7, or choose one from the menu of options.

So, for Days 1-14, I have provided everything for you in an easy-to-follow sequence. And for days 15-30, you may continue with the same system. Start with a Gratitude Grid, choose and complete the suggested Tapping Sequences, and end with writing out a Gratitude List of your choice to complete your meal of assignments.

Frequently Asked Questions

Q: Is the order of assignments important?
A: No, dessert could come first if you prefer! Or you could start with the Tapping Sequence or your Gratitude List and save the Gratitude Grid for the final exercise each day. It's up to you.

Q: What if I don't feel like doing the Gratitude Grid one day?
A: That's up to you. It would be worthwhile to look at why are you having this resistance to doing the Gratitude Grid. The Gratitude Grid will lift your mood 100% of the time. So yes, of course you can skip it, but why would you sabotage yourself this way?

Q: What if I want to make up my own version of the Gratitude List?
A: Great, go for it! I included some of my favorite ones, with the angle I like that pulls more positive ideas out of me. It's up to you.

Q: What happens if I skip an entire day?
A: Go ahead and start counting with Day 1 again, or just pick up where you left off. I believe in not being too rigid, or it ruins the process.

Q: What if new emotions surface? Can I revise or make up my own Tapping Sequences that aren't included in this challenge?
A: Yes of course! I just included my favorite topics for your ease.

Q: I'm new to Tapping, are there basic directions I can follow?

A: Yes, please see directions in Chapter 4, or visit your *Yes, Thank You* book portal at www.theyescode.com/thankyou.

Let's Get Started

- Pick a start date for your 30-Day Gratitude Challenge.
- Each day, start with filling out your Gratitude Grid.
- Each day, complete the Tapping Sequence scheduled for the day. (Or choose one from anywhere in the book that appeals to you.)
- Each day, write out your Gratitude List, or choose one of the sample Gratitude Lists from the menu.

Directions for the Gratitude Grid

Gratitude Grid Work is one of the most powerful exercises I've ever learned from the folks at Abraham-Hicks.com. As far as "bang for the buck" goes, it's exceptional.

I've given you a basic grid to get started, which is simply 16 boxes ready for you to fill in. In each box, write in a word, emotion, or feeling that represents the energy you want to attract for your day. For instance, you could write "Abundance" or "Clarity" or "Peace" or "Joy" or "Fun" or "Stillness" or "Connection" or "Humor" or "Mindfulness" or "Insight" or "Magic" and enjoy raising your vibration.

Gratitude Grid

You can title your Gratitude Grid for separate parts of your life as well. For instance, you could write "Work" at the top of one of your grids, or "Romantic Relationship" and then fill in the boxes with the feelings you would like to experience in relation to the topic you chose.

Tapping Sequences

For Days 1-14, I have provided particularly effective Tapping Sequences with all the phrases typed out for you. I highly recommend starting with what I have provided and then adjust the wording if necessary.

Gratitude Lists

I have provided a number of **Sample Gratitude Lists** for you in both Chapter 10 and at the end of this chapter. I have detailed them below for your first 2 weeks. Use whichever ones you want, and change them according to your mood, or any insights that are revealed to you.

Ready to get started?

DAY #1

Start Day #1 of your Gratitude Challenge by filling out your **Gratitude Grid** for your day, or for a particular part of your life. Then proceed to your daily Tapping Sequences.

Tapping Target #1: I Feel So Overwhelmed

Measure how overwhelmed you feel on the 0-10 point intensity scale.

While tapping on the side of your hand (karate chop point) repeat the setup statements:

Side of Hand: Even though I feel totally overwhelmed, and I can't get clear, I deeply and completely love and accept myself anyway. Even though I feel overwhelmed in my body and mind, I accept and love myself and how I feel.

Now start tapping on the points on the face and body as indicated below:

Eyebrow: I feel so overwhelmed.
Side of Eye: I am deeply overwhelmed.
Under Eye: I am so overwhelmed, I can't be clear.
Under Nose: I can't even think straight.
Chin: I am so overwhelmed.
Collarbone: I really feel overwhelmed.
Under Arm: I am overwhelmed in my body and mind.
Head: I feel so overwhelmed right now.

Take a deep breath, and measure your feeling of overwhelm again on the 0-10 point scale. Either repeat the above Tapping Sequence focused on your target issue, or proceed to the Gratitude Tapping I've outlined for you below.

Side of Hand: Even though I still feel overwhelmed, I deeply and completely love and accept myself anyway. Even though I still feel so overwhelmed, I accept who I am and how I feel.
Eyebrow: I feel grateful I recognize what I'm going through.
Side of Eye: Thank you for validating my feelings.

Under Eye: I appreciate all that I have learned.
Under Nose: I appreciate that I am ok right now.
Chin: Thank you for helping me feel better already.
Collarbone: Thank you, Universe, for bringing me a solution.
Under Arm: Thank you, Universe, for solving this issue for me.
Head: Thank you, Universe, for helping me release my overwhelm.

Take another deep breath, and measure how overwhelmed you feel now on the 0-10 point scale. Repeat the Gratitude Tapping as many times as you wish.

Next, write out your Gratitude List. Use the one I provide here, one from Chapter 10, or choose another one from the sample list at the end of this chapter.

<u>**Gratitude List:**</u> 10 Things I love About My Life.

_____

_____

_____

_____

_____

_____

_____

_____

_____

_____

DAY #2

Start Day #2 of your Gratitude Challenge by filling out a **Gratitude Grid**. Then proceed to your daily Tapping Sequences.

Tapping Target #2: I Feel So Stressed Out

Measure how stressed you feel on the 0-10 point intensity scale. While tapping on the side of your hand or karate chop point, repeat the setup statements.

Side of Hand: Even though I feel totally stressed out, I deeply and completely love and accept myself right now. Even though I feel completely stressed out in my body and mind, I accept and love myself anyway.

Now use the Tapping Sequence below:

Eyebrow: I feel so stressed out.
Side of Eye: I have so much stress in my life.
Under Eye: I have so much stress everywhere.
Under Nose: I am very stressed out.
Chin: I'm not handling my stress very well.
Collarbone: I wish I didn't react so much.
Under Arm: I feel so much stress every day.
Head: I feel stress in every part of my life.

Take a deep breath and measure your stress level on the 0-10 point scale again. You may repeat the above Tapping Sequence or proceed to the Gratitude Tapping listed below.

Side of Hand: Even though I still feel so stressed out, I deeply and completely love and accept myself. Even though I still have so much stress in my life, I accept who I am and how I feel.

Eyebrow: I am grateful I feel better already.
Side of Eye: I'm learning to handle stress with more grace.
Under Eye: I appreciate what the Universe is teaching me.
Under Nose: Thank you, Universe, for so many lessons about myself.
Chin: Thank you, Universe, for resolving this issue for me.

Collarbone: Thank you, Universe, for delivering a solution.
Under Arm: Thank you for all that I'm learning.
Head: I am so grateful that I feel better already.

Take a deep breath, and measure your stress level again on the 0-10 point scale.

Repeat the Gratitude Tapping Sequence as many times as you wish. When you're ready, proceed to your Gratitude List.

<u>**Gratitude List:**</u> 10 things that make me feel good.

_____

_____

_____

_____

_____

_____

_____

_____

_____

_____

DAY #3

Start Day #3 of your Gratitude Challenge by filling out your **Gratitude Grid**. Then proceed to your Tapping Sequences for the day.

Tapping Target #3: I Don't Trust My Inner Voice

Measure how true this statement feels to you on the 0-10 point intensity scale.

While tapping on the side of your hand (karate chop point), repeat the setup statements:

Side of Hand: Even though I don't trust my inner voice, I choose to appreciate that it is always there for me. Even though I am afraid of trusting my inner voice, I accept and love myself and how I feel.

Now use the Tapping Sequence as indicated below:

Eyebrow: I don't trust my inner voice.
Side of Eye: I'm afraid to trust my inner voice.
Under Eye: I'm not in the habit of trusting my inner voice.
Under Nose: I ignore it all the time.
Chin: I ignore my inner voice out of habit.
Collarbone: I don't trust that it knows what I need.
Under Arm: I'm afraid to make a mistake.
Head: I don't trust my inner voice.

Take a deep breath, and measure your fear of trusting your inner voice again on the 0-10 point scale. Either repeat the above Tapping Sequence, or proceed to the Thank You Tapping listed below.

Side of Hand: Even though I still don't trust my inner voice, I deeply and completely love and accept myself anyway. Even though I still don't trust my inner voice, what if it's wrong, I deeply and completely love and accept myself now.

Eyebrow: Thank you, Universe, for letting me trust myself.
Side of Eye: Thank you, Universe, for releasing this fear.

Under Eye: Thank you, Universe, for so many blessings.
Under Nose: I love listening to my inner voice.
Chin: I appreciate my inner voice, thank you.
Collarbone: I appreciate my inner guidance.
Under Arm: I love that I can trust my inner guidance.
Head: Thank you, Universe, for my inner guidance.

Take a deep breath, and measure your fear of trusting your inner voice again on the 0-10 point scale. Repeat the Thank You Tapping Sequence as many times as you wish.

Then proceed to your daily Gratitude List.

<u>**Gratitude List**</u>**:** I feel grateful whenever these 10 things happen.

_____

_____

_____

_____

_____

_____

_____

_____

_____

_____

DAY #4

Start Day #4 by filling out your **Gratitude Grid**. Then proceed to your daily Tapping Sequences.

Tapping Target #4: I Feel Emotional Clutter in My Mind

If possible, measure how emotionally cluttered you feel or how much distress you feel about having emotional clutter on the 0-10 point intensity scale.

While tapping your side of the hand, repeat the setup statements:

Side of Hand: Even though I feel totally cluttered in my mind, and it's annoying, I deeply and completely love and accept myself anyway. Even though I feel cluttered with too many conflicts and emotions in my mind, I accept and love myself and how I feel.

Now proceed to the Tapping Sequence below:

Eyebrow: I feel emotional clutter.
Side of Eye: I feel so unclear.
Under Eye: I feel emotional clutter.
Under Nose: I feel so many conflicts and so much clutter.
Chin: There are so many emotional conflicts.
Collarbone: I have so much emotional clutter.
Under Arm: I feel so much emotional clutter.
Head: It's upsetting to feel so cluttered in my mind.

Measure the distress you feel about your emotional clutter on the 0-10 point scale again. Either repeat the above Tapping Sequence or proceed to the Gratitude Tapping listed below.

Side of Hand: Even though I still feel so much emotional clutter, I deeply and completely love and accept myself. Even though I still feel so many emotional conflicts and clutter, I deeply and completely love and accept myself.

Eyebrow: I appreciate the emotions I do have.

Side of Eye: I appreciate the solution the Universe has sent me.
Under Eye: I appreciate that I recognize the challenges.
Under Nose: I appreciate what I've learned.
Chin: I appreciate my mind no matter what.
Collarbone: I appreciate so much about my mind.
Under Arm: I appreciate everything that I feel.
Head: Thank you for all my emotions.

Repeat the Gratitude Tapping Sequence as many times as you wish. Then proceed to your Gratitude List using the topic I provide below, or choose another one from the sample list at the end of this chapter.

<u>Gratitude List</u>: I love it when…(list 10 things).

_____

_____

_____

_____

_____

_____

_____

_____

_____

_____

DAY #5

Start Day #5 of your Gratitude Challenge by filling out your **Gratitude Grid**. Then proceed to your daily Tapping Sequences.

Tapping Target #5: I'm Afraid of Being Clear

Measure how afraid you feel of being clear on the 0-10 point intensity scale.

While tapping on the side of your hand, repeat the setup statements:

Side of Hand: Even though I feel afraid to be clear, no wonder I sabotage myself, I deeply and completely love and accept myself anyway. Even though I feel afraid to be clear about my decisions, I accept and love myself and how I feel.

Eyebrow: I'm afraid to be clear.
Side of Eye: There might be negative consequences.
Under Eye: I'm afraid to be clear.
Under Nose: I don't want to take a stand.
Chin: I'm afraid to make a commitment.
Collarbone: I'm so afraid to be clear.
Under Arm: No wonder I sabotage my success.
Head: I'm afraid to be clear and move forward.

Take a deep breath and measure your fear of being clear again on the 0-10 point scale. Either repeat the above Tapping Sequence or proceed to the Gratitude Tapping listed below.

Side of Hand: Even though a part of me is still afraid to be clear, I deeply and profoundly love and accept myself anyway. Even though there's still a part of me that's afraid to make a commitment, I accept who I am and how I feel.

Eyebrow: I'm grateful that I'm aware that I'm afraid.
Side of Eye: I'm grateful that I know what's going on.
Under Eye: I'm grateful that I know what's in my way.
Under Nose: Thank you, Universe, for pointing this out.

Chin: Thank you, Universe, for sending me a solution.
Collarbone: Thank you, Universe, for so much validation.
Under Arm: Thank you, Universe, for so much acknowledgment.
Head: Thank you, Universe, for clearing my fears.

Repeat the Gratitude Tapping as many times as you wish. Then complete the Gratitude List I provide below or choose one from the menu of options at the end of this section.

<u>**Gratitude List:**</u> I appreciate the following 10 people in my life.

_____

_____

_____

_____

_____

_____

_____

_____

_____

_____

DAY #6

Start Day #6 of your Gratitude Challenge by completing your **Gratitude Grid** on any topic. Then proceed to your daily Tapping Sequences.

Tapping Target #6: I'm Afraid to Shine

Measure your fear of shining on the 0-10 point intensity scale. While tapping on the side of your hand, repeat the setup statements.

Side of Hand: Even though I feel afraid to shine, I deeply and completely love and accept myself anyway. Even though I feel afraid to shine in my life, I accept and love myself and how I feel.

Eyebrow: I'm afraid to shine.
Side of Eye: I don't like the attention.
Under Eye: I'm afraid to shine.
Under Nose: I don't want to be noticed.
Chin: It doesn't feel safe to me.
Collarbone: I'm afraid to shine.
Under Arm: I don't want to be visible.
Head: It feels safer to stay under the radar.

Take a deep breath, and measure your fear of shining again on the 0-10 point scale. Either repeat the above phrases or proceed to the Gratitude Tapping listed below.

Side of Hand: Even though I'm still afraid to shine and be noticed, I deeply and profoundly love and accept myself anyway. Even though I'm still afraid to shine because I don't want to be visible, I accept who I am and how I feel.

Eyebrow: I'm so grateful I know what the problem is.
Side of Eye: I'm grateful for all that I have in my life.
Under eye: I'm grateful even if I'm afraid to shine.
Under Nose: Thank you, Universe, for so much success.
Chin: Thank you, Universe, for all the blessings I have.
Collarbone: I'm grateful for so much abundance in my life.
Under Arm: Thank you, Universe, for so many blessings.

Head: I'm grateful for how blessed I feel.

Repeat the Gratitude Tapping Sequence as many times as you wish. Then proceed to writing out your Gratitude List.

Gratitude List: I appreciate these 10 blessings in my life.

_____

_____

_____

_____

_____

_____

_____

_____

DAY #7

Start Day #7 of your Gratitude Challenge by completing your **Gratitude Grid**. Then proceed to your daily Tapping Sequences.

Tapping Target #7: Fear of Success

Measure how afraid of success you feel on the 0-10 point intensity scale.

While tapping on the side of your hand, repeat the setup statements.

Side of Hand: Even though I feel afraid to be successful, I deeply and completely love and accept myself anyway. Even though I feel afraid of how success might change me, I accept and love myself and how I feel now.

Eyebrow: I'm afraid of success.
Side of Eye: I'm afraid to succeed.
Under Eye: I'm not sure I can handle it.
Under Nose: I'm afraid of success.
Chin: I'm afraid I can't handle it.
Collarbone: I'm afraid I won't be able to handle it.
Under Arm: I'm afraid of what success might do to my life.
Head: I'm afraid to be successful.

Take a deep breath and measure your fear of success again on the 0-10 point scale. Either repeat the above Tapping Phrases or proceed to the Gratitude Tapping listed below.

Side of Hand: Even though I'm afraid to succeed, I'm not sure I can handle it, I deeply and profoundly love and accept myself. Even though I'm afraid of what success might do to my life, I deeply and profoundly love and accept myself anyway.

Eyebrow: I'm grateful for the success I have had.
Side of Eye: I'm grateful for what I do have in my life.
Under Eye: I'm grateful I'm figuring this out now.
Under Nose: I'm grateful for so much in my life.
Chin: Thank you, Universe, for so many blessings.
Collarbone: Thank you, Universe, for so much abundance.

Under Arm: I love all the abundance in my life.
Head: Thank you, Universe, for all the success I already have.

Take a deep breath, and measure your fear of success again on the 0-10 point scale. Repeat the Gratitude Tapping Sequence as many times as you wish. Then proceed to your Gratitude List.

<u>**Gratitude List**</u>: I love counting my many blessings, especially...(list 10 things).

_____

_____

_____

_____

_____

_____

_____

_____

_____

_____

Congratulations! You've completed the first week of your 30-Day Gratitude Challenge.

DAY #8

Start Day #8 of your Gratitude Challenge by filling out your **Gratitude Grid**. Then proceed to your daily Tapping Sequences.

Tapping Target #8: I Feel So Impatient

Measure how impatient you feel on the 0-10 point intensity scale. You could be focused on a job opportunity, abundance coming in too slowly, on a relationship, or anything else that you feel impatient about.

While tapping on your side of the hand, repeat the following setup statements.

Side of Hand: Even though I feel impatient that my abundance hasn't shown up yet, I deeply and completely love and accept myself anyway. Even though I feel impatient because I'm doing everything I'm supposed to do and it still hasn't shown up for me, I accept and love myself and how I feel.

Eyebrow: I feel so impatient that my abundance isn't here yet.
Side of Eye: Why isn't it here yet?
Under eye: I've done everything I'm supposed to do.
Under Nose: I feel so impatient.
Chin: Hurry up, Universe!
Collarbone: Why aren't I being rewarded?
Under Arm: I'm really impatient about it.
Head: Part of me wants to give up.

Take a deep breath, and measure your level of impatience again on the 0-10 point scale. Either repeat the above Tapping Sequence or proceed to the Gratitude Tapping below.

Side of Hand: Even though I still feel so impatient that my abundance isn't here yet, I deeply and completely love and accept myself. Even though I still feel so impatient that my abundance hasn't arrived yet, I accept who I am and how I feel.

Eyebrow: The truth is I already have a lot of abundance.
Side of Eye: The truth is I already see some results.

Under Eye: I'm impatient about everything.
Under Nose: Thank you, Universe, for bringing me so much abundance.
Chin: Thank you, Universe, for the abundance that I do have.
Collarbone: Thank you, Universe, for so many blessings.
Under Arm: Thank you, Universe, for teaching me so much.
Head: Thank you, Universe, for all the blessings I have.

Take a deep breath and measure your impatience again on the 0-10 point scale. Repeat the Gratitude Tapping as many times as you wish. Then proceed to your Gratitude List below.

<u>**Gratitude List**</u>: I love it when...(10 things).

_____
_____
_____
_____
_____
_____
_____
_____
_____
_____

DAY #9

Start Day #9 of your challenge by filling in your **Gratitude Grid**. Then proceed to the Tapping Sequences below.

Tapping Target #9: I'm Afraid to Be Quiet

Measure how afraid you feel of being quiet on the 0-10 point intensity scale.

While tapping on the side of your hand or karate chop point, repeat the setup statements.

Side of Hand: Even though I'm afraid to be still and quiet, and I know that blocks my abundance, I deeply and completely love and accept myself anyway. Even though I feel afraid to be quiet and still in my body in mind, I accept and love myself and how I feel.

Eyebrow: I'm afraid to be quiet.
Side of Eye: It makes me nervous.
Under Eye: I'm afraid of what I might feel.
Under Nose: I feel safer when I'm distracted.
Chin: It's hard to be still and quiet.
Collarbone: I'm afraid of what emotions might surface.
Under Arm: I'm afraid to be quiet.
Head: I'd rather be too busy.

Take a deep breath and measure your fear of being quiet again on the 0-10 point scale. Either repeat the above Tapping Sequence or proceed to the Gratitude Tapping listed below.

Side of Hand: Even though I'm still afraid to be quiet, I deeply and completely love and accept myself anyway. Even though I'm still afraid of what I might feel, I deeply and completely love and accept myself anyway.

Eyebrow: I'm grateful that I know how to be quiet.
Side of Eye: I'm grateful that I'm stretching my capacity.
Under Eye: I'm grateful it's OK for me to be afraid.
Under Nose: Thank you, Universe, for all the blessings in my life.

Chin: What if being quiet is a good thing?
Collarbone: I appreciate that being quiet would be good for me.
Under Arm: I appreciate that being quiet is soothing.
Head: Thank you, Universe, for teaching me about being quiet.

Take a deep breath, and measure your fear of being quiet again on the 0-10 point scale. Repeat the Gratitude Tapping Sequence as many times as you wish.

Now proceed to filling out your Gratitude List.

Gratitude List: 10 things I love about my life.

_____

_____

_____

_____

_____

_____

_____

_____

_____

_____

DAY #10

Start Day #10 by filling out your **Gratitude Grid**. Then proceed with today's Tapping Sequences.

Tapping Target #10: I'm Conflicted About Success

If possible, measure how conflicted you feel about your success on the 0-10 point intensity scale. While tapping on the side of your hand, repeat the setup statements.

Side of Hand: Even though I feel conflicted about my success, I deeply and completely love and accept myself anyway. Even though a part of me wants to be successful, and another part does not, I deeply and completely love and accept myself anyway.

Eyebrow: I feel so conflicted about success.
Side of Eye: A part of me wants to be successful.
Under Eye: A part of me is afraid I will fail.
Under Nose: I'm so conflicted about my success.
Chin: I don't want to commit to success.
Collarbone: I'm so conflicted by success.
Under Arm: No wonder I'm not aligned with it.
Head: I'm afraid to go all in with success.

Take a deep breath, and measure your level of conflict about being successful again on the 0-10 point scale. Either repeat the above Tapping Sequence or proceed to the Gratitude Tapping below:

Side of Hand: Even though I'm still conflicted about my success, I deeply and completely love and accept myself. Even though I still feel conflicted about my success, I accept who I am and how I feel.

Eyebrow: I appreciate that I am honoring my feelings.
Side of Eye: I appreciate that all my feelings are valid.
Under Eye: I am grateful for this conflict.
Under Nose: It's teaching me a lot about my desires.
Chin: I'm grateful for so much in my life.
Collarbone: I appreciate that this conflict is instructive.

Under Arm: Thank you, Universe, for allowing me to have my feelings.
Head: Thank you, Universe, for the lessons from this conflict.

Take a deep breath and measure your conflict about success again on the 0-10 point scale.

Repeat the Gratitude Tapping Sequence as many times as you wish and then proceed to writing out your Gratitude List. You may choose one of the lists from Chapter 10, from Gratitude List Options at the end of this chapter, or come up with your own.

DAY #11

Start Day #11 of your Gratitude Challenge by filling out your **Gratitude Grid**. Then proceed to your daily Tapping Sequences below.

Tapping Target #11: I Feel Exhausted and Fatigued

Measure how exhausted you feel on the 0-10 point intensity scale. While tapping on the side of your hand, repeat the setup statements.

Side of Hand: Even though I feel totally exhausted and fatigued, so I can't even focus on gratitude, I deeply and completely love and accept myself anyway. Even though I feel so tired and exhausted in my body and mind, I accept and love myself and how I feel.

Eyebrow: I feel exhausted and fatigued.
Side of Eye: I feel so tired, deep down.
Under Eye: I feel so tired and exhausted.
Under Nose: I ran myself into the ground.
Chin: I'm so exhausted, I can't focus on gratitude.
Collarbone: I've overworked again, so I forget my gratitude.
Under Arm: I'm so tired, I can't focus on gratitude.
Head: I'm so exhausted and fatigued.

Take a deep breath and measure your level of exhaustion again on the 0-10 point scale. Either repeat the above Tapping Phrases or proceed to the Gratitude Tapping Sequence below.

Side of Hand: Even though I'm still tired and exhausted, and it gets in the way of my gratitude, I deeply and completely love and accept myself. Even though I'm still tired and exhausted, and it interferes with my gratitude, I accept who I am and how I feel.

Eyebrow: I'm grateful that I'm starting to feel better.
Side of Eye: I feel grateful for my body anyway.
Under Eye: Thank you, Universe, for so much abundance in my life.
Under Nose: I love so many things about my body.
Chin: Thank you, Universe, for so many blessings in my life.
Collarbone: I appreciate so much in my life.

Under Arm: Thank you, Universe, for my strength.
Head: I am grateful for what I am able to do.

Take a deep breath, and measure your level of fatigue again on the 0-10 point scale. Repeat the Gratitude Tapping Sequence as many times as you wish, and then proceed to your Gratitude List.

Gratitude List: Count your blessings, at least 10 of them (or choose one of the Gratitude Lists detailed in Chapter 10, or at the end of this section).

_____
_____
_____
_____
_____
_____
_____
_____
_____
_____

DAY #12

Start Day #12 of your Gratitude Challenge by filling in your **Gratitude Grid**. You may focus on what you want to feel for the day, or focus on a particular part of your life. Then proceed to your daily Tapping Sequences below.

Tapping Target #12: I Ignore My Blessings

Sometimes we all ignore our blessings. Measure how true this is for you or how guilty you feel about it on the 0-10 point intensity scale.

While tapping on the side of your hand, repeat the setup statements.

Side of Hand: Even though I sometimes ignore the blessings in my life, I choose to appreciate how many I have. Even though I tend to ignore all the blessings in my life, and I feel guilty about it, I accept and love myself anyway.

Eyebrow: I ignore my blessings sometimes.
Side of Eye: I tend to ignore my blessings.
Under Eye: I sometimes ignore my blessings.
Under Nose: I ignore my blessings regularly.
Chin: I feel guilty when I ignore my blessings.
Collarbone: I wish I noticed more of my blessings.
Under Arm: I don't notice my blessings frequently enough.
Head: Sometimes I ignore my blessings.

Take a deep breath, and measure how true this feels to you now on the 0-10 point scale, or how guilty you feel about it. Either repeat the above Tapping Sequence, or proceed to the Thank You Tapping below.

Side of Hand: Even though I still have a bad habit of ignoring my blessings, I deeply and profoundly love and accept myself. Even though I still ignore my blessings sometimes, I accept who I am and how I feel.

Eyebrow: Thank you, Universe, for letting me notice my blessings.
Side of Eye: Thank you, Universe, for helping me with this issue.
Under Eye: Thank you, Universe, for so many blessings.
Under Nose: I love noticing all the blessings in my life.

Chin: Thank you, Universe, I appreciate all the blessings in my life.
Collarbone: I appreciate that I notice all my blessings.
Under Arm: I love all the blessings in my life.
Head: I appreciate all my blessings.

Take a deep breath, and measure how true this feels to you now on the 0-10 point scale. Check whether your guilt has decreased about this topic.

Now fill out your Gratitude List for the day, or count your blessings.

Gratitude List: 10 things I appreciate about myself.

_____
_____
_____
_____
_____
_____
_____
_____
_____
_____

DAY #13

Start Day #13 of your Gratitude Challenge by filling in your **Gratitude Grid**. Then proceed to the Tapping Sequences for today.

Tapping Target #13: I'm Afraid to Slow Down

Measure how afraid you feel of slowing down on the 0-10 point intensity scale. If possible, identify why you feel afraid of slowing down. While tapping on the side of your hand, repeat the setup statements.

Side of Hand: Even though I'm afraid to slow down because I might feel empty or lonely, I deeply and completely love and accept myself. Even though I'm afraid to slow down because I'm not sure what emotions might surface, I choose to accept myself and my feelings.

Eyebrow: I'm afraid to slow down.
Side of Eye: I'm afraid I might feel too much.
Under Eye: No wonder I'm always busy.
Under Nose: I'm afraid to slow down.
Chin: I don't want to feel empty or lonely.
Collarbone: I'm afraid to slow down.
Under Arm: I'm afraid of what I might feel.
Head: No wonder I won't slow down.

Take a breath and measure your fear of slowing down again on the 0-10 point scale. Repeat the above Tapping Phrases or proceed to the Gratitude Tapping Sequence below.

Side of Hand: Even though I'm still afraid of slowing down, what if I feel too many feelings, I deeply and completely love and accept myself. Even though I'm afraid to slow down, what if I feel too much, I accept who I am and how I feel.

Eyebrow: Thank you, Universe, for showing me how to slow down.
Side of Eye: Thank you, Universe, for helping me slow down.
Under Eye: Thank you, Universe, for so many blessings in my life.
Under Nose: What if slowing down will be good for me?
Chin: What if slowing down will help me feel grateful?

Collarbone: Thank you, Universe, for showing me the truth.
Under Arm: I'm grateful for what I've learned.
Head: Thank you, Universe, for sending me so many solutions.

Take a deep breath and measure your fear of slowing down again on the 0-10 point scale. Repeat the Gratitude Tapping as many times as you wish. Then proceed to writing your Gratitude List.

<u>**Gratitude List**</u>: 10 things I appreciate about my body.

_____
_____
_____
_____
_____
_____
_____
_____
_____
_____

DAY #14

Start Day #14 by filling out your <u>**Gratitude Grid.**</u> Then move on to the Tapping Sequences for today.

Tapping Target #14: I Feel Resistant to Change

Measure your resistance to change on the 0-10 point intensity scale. While tapping the side of your hand repeat the setup statements below.

Side of Hand: Even though I feel resistant to change, I deeply and completely love and accept myself anyway. Even though I'm afraid to change, I accept all of me anyway.

Eyebrow: I'm so resistant to change.
Side of Eye: I'm afraid to make deep changes.
Under Eye: I can feel my resistance right now.
Under Nose: I can really feel my resistance now.
Chin: I feel resistant to change.
Collarbone: I'm afraid to get better.
Under Arm: I don't like how my resistance feels.
Head: I don't want to change.

Take a deep breath, and measure your resistance or fear of change again on the 0-10 point scale.

Either repeat the above Tapping Sequence or proceed to the Thank You Tapping listed below.

Side of Hand: Even though I feel so resistant to change, I deeply and completely love and accept myself. Even though I feel so afraid of change, I deeply and completely love and accept myself.

Eyebrow: Thank you, Universe, for helping me release my resistance.
Side of Eye: Thank you, Universe, for showing me what to do next.
Under Eye: Thank you, Universe, for helping me move forward.
Under Nose: I love feeling free of resistance.
Chin: I appreciate that it's time to release some of my resistance.
Collarbone: I appreciate my fear of changing.

Under Arm: Thank you, Universe, for all my emotions.

Head: I appreciate every part of me, even my resistance.

Take a deep breath, and measure your fear and resistance of change again on the 0-10 point scale. Repeat the Gratitude Tapping as many times as you wish. Then proceed to one of the Gratitude Lists of your choice.

<u>**Gratitude List:**</u> I'm so grateful for these blessings in my life (list 10 things).

_____

_____

_____

_____

_____

_____

_____

_____

_____

_____

Congratulations! You have completed another week of your 30-Day Gratitude Challenge.

What's Next?

DAYS #15 - #30

1. For the next 14 days, the structure is the same. Please start each day by filling out a **Gratitude Grid**. You may choose any of the options from the list at the end of this chapter.

2. Then complete a **Tapping Sequence** for each day. You may repeat one of the Tapping Sequences from the first 14 days, choose one of the sequences from Chapters 5-8, or choose one from the Tapping Target Options below.

3. Finally, finish off each day of your Gratitude Challenge with a **Gratitude List**. You may use one of the Gratitude Invitations or practices I describe in Chapter 10, choose one from the first 14 days, or choose a list from the **Gratitude List Options** below.

Congratulations! Now You Have Completed your 30-Day Gratitude Challenge!

I highly recommend that you journal about your experience.

And then...

Start again!

Below I have detailed options for your Gratitude Grid, your Tapping Targets, and your Gratitude Lists.

Gratitude Grid Options

You may "name" your grid according to any part of your life you would like to focus on for this exercise.

1. My life
2. My day
3. My work
4. Professional opportunities
5. My romantic relationship
6. My past
7. My family

Yes, Thank You • 215

8. My future
9. My health

Tapping Target Options

While there are dozens of Tapping Targets throughout Part 3 of the book and in the first 14 days of the Gratitude Challenge, I have added some more options below.

1. There's not enough for me.
2. I feel anxious all the time.
3. I'm worried I'm doing this wrong.
4. I'm afraid of being myself.
5. I'm afraid they'll reject me.
6. I'm convinced I'll push them away.
7. I'm afraid I'm not enough.
8. I'm afraid I don't have what it takes.
9. I'm afraid I'm not smart enough.
10. I'm afraid it's too late.

Gratitude List Options

There are numerous Gratitude Lists and practices detailed in Chapter 10, and in the first 14 days of this challenge. Choose one of those or one of the ones below.

1. 10 things I love about my life.
2. 10 things that make me feel good.
3. I feel grateful whenever these 10 things happen.
4. I love it when…
5. I appreciate the following 10 people in my life.
6. I appreciate the following 10 things in my life.
7. I love all these blessings in my life.
8. I'm grateful that these things happened in my past.
9. I love the following things about my body.
10. I appreciate the following characteristics about me.

Scan this QR code or visit your *Yes, Thank You* book portal at www.theyescode.com/thankyou for a downloadable and printable copy of the 30-Day Gratitude Challenge.

Conclusion

If I had started using EFT at an early age, I would have cleared my blocks and started and stuck to a gratitude practice earlier in my life. Instead, I took a long and winding path, and I'm grateful I have the tools now.

There are self-help tools, and then there is EFT Tapping, the exquisite emotional technology that can change your life as soon as you pick it up.

There are powerful self-care practices, and then there is expressing gratitude, the superpower of all superpowers.

In a survey about which superpower people most wanted, the highest number of participants responded with wanting the superpower "to heal others" and the second most popular response was "to fly."[34]

Expressing gratitude on a regular basis won't help you heal others or fly, but it will help you improve all other parts of your life.

My wish for you after reading this book is that you feel inspired to combine EFT Tapping and a daily gratitude practice to achieve exponential results and enjoy the life you were meant to live.

I feel so grateful to be on this path with you all. We are certainly in it together.

With many thanks,
Carol Look, LCSW, Founding EFT Master

Endnotes

Introduction

1. Mary Oliver, "The Summer Day," *Library of Congress*, 1990, https://www.loc.gov/programs/poetry-and-literature/poet-laureate/poet-laureate-projects/poetry-180/all-poems/item/poetry-180-133/the-summer-day/.

2. Robert A. Emmons, *Thanks!: How the New Science of Gratitude Can Make You Happier*, (Houghton Mifflin Co. 2007), 27.

3. Anna L. Boggiss, Nathan S. Consedine, Jennifer M. Brenton-Peters, Paul L. Hofman, and Anna S. Serlachius, "A Systematic Review of Gratitude Interventions: Effects on Physical Health and Health Behaviors," *Journal of Psychosomatic Research* 135 (1) (2020), https://doi.org/10.1016/j.jpsychores.2020.110165.

4. Emmons, *Thanks*, 30.

5. Abdul Basit, Ramzan Ali, Summiya Rahman, and Aizaz Ali Shah, "Exploring How the Practice of Gratitude Can Strengthen Interpersonal Relationships, Enhance Mental Well-Being, Foster Emotional Resilience, and Promote Greater Social Connectedness and Cooperation," *Review of Education Administration and Law* 7 (4) (2024): 427–41. https://doi.org/10.47067/real.v7i4.395.

6. Joe Dispenza, "The Power of Gratitude," *Dr. Joe Dispenza*, 2016, https://drjoedispenza.com/dr-joes-blog/the-power-of-gratitude.

7. Eri Eguchi, Kokoro Shirai, Fumikazu Hayazhi, Yuhi Hamaguchi, Katsunori Kondo, and Tetsuya Ohira, "Abstract P230: Association between Gratitude and Lifestyle Related Diseases: The JAGES Cross-Sectional Study," *Circulation* 149 (Suppl_1) (2024): https://doi.org/10.1161/circ.149.suppl_1.p230.

8. Geyze Diniz, Ligia Korkes, Luca Schiliró Tristão, Rosangela Pelegrini, Patrícia Lacerda Bellodi, and Wanderley Marques Bernardo, "The Effects of Gratitude Interventions: A Systematic Review and Meta-Analysis," *Einstein Journal (São Paulo)* 21 (2023): https://doi.org/10.31744/einstein_journal/2023rw0371.

9. Najma Khorrami, "Gratitude Helps Minimize Feelings of Stress," *Psychology Today*, 2020, https://www.psychologytoday.com/us/blog/comfort-gratitude/202007/gratitude-helps-minimize-feelings-stress?.

10. Susan Kreimer, "Living Longer Tied to Gratitude for Positives in Life, Harvard Study Suggests," *UPI*, July 3, 2024, https://www.upi.com/Health_News/2024/07/03/uslive-longer-gratitude/4471720016598/.

11. David Speigel, MD, "Living Longer Tied to Gratitude for Positives in Life, Harvard Study Suggests," *UPI*, July 3, 2024, https://www.upi.com/Health_News/2024/07/03/uslive-longer-gratitude/4471720016598/.

12. Linda A Baker, "Can Gratitude Improve Quality of Life?," *Princeton Health News*, 2023, https://www.princetonhcs.org/about-princeton-health/news-and-information/news/can-gratitude-increase-quality-of-life.

13. Amanda Cross, "26 Employee Recognition Statistics You Need to Know in 2024," *Nectar*, 2024, https://nectarhr.com/blog/employee-recognition-statistics?.

14. Brené Brown, "I Don't Have to Chase Extraordinary Moments to Find Happiness--It's Right in Front of Me," *Forbes,* July 15, 2011, https://www.forbes.com/sites/gretchenrubin/2011/07/15/i-dont-have-to-chase-extraordinary-moments-to-find-hapiness-its-right-in-front-of-me/.

15. Eguchi et al, "Association Between Gratitude."

16. "Suicide Data and Statistics," *CDC*, October 29, 2024, https://www.cdc.gov/suicide/facts/data.html.

17. Melinda Ratini, "The Effects of Stress on Your Body," *WebMD*, February 2007, https://www.webmd.com/balance/stress-management/effects-of-stress-on-your-body.

Chapter 2

18. Oprah Winfrey, *What I Know for Sure*, (Flatiron Books, 2014).

Chapter 4

19. Donna Bach, Gary Groesbeck, Peta Stapleton, Rebecca Sims, Katharina Blickheuser, and Dawson Church, "Clinical EFT (Emotional Freedom Techniques) Improves Multiple Physiological Markers of Health," *Journal of Evidence-Based Integrative Medicine* 24 (January 1, 2019): https://doi.org/10.1177/2515690x18823691.

20. Peta Stapleton, Craig Buchan, Ian Mitchell, Yasmin McGrath, Paul Gorton & Brett Carter, "An Initial Investigation of Neural Changes in Overweight Adults with Food Cravings after Emotional Freedom Techniques," *OBM Integrative and Complementary Medicine* 4, no 1 (2019): https://doi.org/10.21926/obm.icm.1901010.

21. P.B. Stapleton, O. Baumann, T. O'Keefe, and S. Bhuta, "Neural Changes After Emotional Freedom Techniques Treatment for Chronic Pain Sufferers," *Complementary Therapies in Clinical Practice* 49 (November 2022): https://doi.org/10.1016/j.ctcp.2022.101653.

22. Peta Stapleton, PhD, *The Science Behind Tapping: A Proven Stress Management Technique for the Mind and Body* (Hay House, Inc., 2022).

23. David Feinstein and Donna Eden, *Tapping: Self-Healing with the Transformative Power of Energy Psychology*, (Sounds True, 2024).

24. Stapleton, *The Science Behind Tapping*.

25. Feinstein and Eden, *Tapping*.

Chapter 5

26. "Kübler-Ross Change Curve®," *Elizabeth Kubler-Ross Foundation*, August 5, 2024, https://www.ekrfoundation.org/5-stages-of-grief/change-curve/#:~:text=Elisabeth%20Kübler%2DRoss%20introduced%20the,change%2C%20loss%2C%20or%20shock.

Chapter 6

27. Jennifer Guttman, Psy.D., "The Relationship with Yourself," *Psychology Today*, June 27, 2019, https://www.psychologytoday.com/ca/blog/sustainable-life-satisfaction/201906/the-relationship-yourself.

Chapter 7

28. Dena M. Bravata, Sharon A. Watts, Autumn L. Keefer, Divya K. Madhusudhan, Katie T. Taylor, Dani M. Clark, Ross S. Nelson, Kevin O. Cokley, and Heather K, Hagg, "Prevalence, Predictors, and Treatment of Impostor Syndrome: A Systematic Review," *Journal of General Internal Medicine* (April 2020): https://pmc.ncbi.nlm.nih.gov/articles/PMC7174434/.

Chapter 8

29. "The Facts about Migraine," *American Migraine Foundation*, March 28, 2019, https://americanmigrainefoundation.org/resource-library/migraine-facts/.

30. "What Are Autoimmune Diseases?," *Cleveland Clinic*, February 8, 2025, https://my.clevelandclinic.org/health/diseases/21624-autoimmune-diseases.

31. "Get Autoimmune Disorders Treatment," *Cleveland Clinic*, Accessed March 18, 2025, https://my.clevelandclinic.org/services/autoimmune-disorders-treatment.

Chapter 10

32. Robert A. Emmons, *Gratitude Works!: A Twenty-One-Day Program For Creating Emotional Prosperity* (Jossey-Bass, 2013), 11.

Chapter 11

33. Eckhart Tolle, *A New Earth: Awakening to Your Life's Purpose,* (Dutton/Penguin Group, 1948-2005), 190.

Conclusion

34. "United States - Preferred Super Powers of Americans in 2018," *Statista,* April 2018, https://www.statista.com/statistics/832262/preferred-super-powers-of-americans/.

Gratitude

I would like to express my deepest appreciation to all my clients, past and present, who taught me the real meaning of gratitude.

Many thanks to Sara Connell, Jane Ubell-Meyer, and the team at Thought Leader Academy Publishing for supporting another dream and ushering this book through to the end. Special thanks to Claudine Mansour for another fabulous cover.

To my editor, Mary Balice Nelligan: What a journey. You did it again! Thank you for your patience, your clarity, and for keeping me on track with my message. You are an exceptionally talented editor, and I'm so grateful we were paired up together.

To Dana Pemberton: It would be hard to use enough words to express my gratitude for all you did to support me through this process this year. Your wisdom, patience, and brilliant guidance made all the difference in keeping me on my path.

To Colleen Robinson: Once again, I roped you in at the last minute. A million thanks for your research, your dedication to detail, and your compassion that pushed this book over the finish line on time. Your emotional intelligence is incredible.

To Rick Wilkes: Thank you for always having my back, and for your attention to detail, your support of all my visions, and your impeccable integrity. I definitely couldn't have done this without you.

To my friends: Leslie Vellios, Heidi Garis, John Cisternino, Peta Stapleton, Michèle Stoudmann, Roos van der Blom, Alissa Smith, Christina Nylese, Carissa Brockman, Dawn Elgin, Julie Fedeli, Yuberka Cabrera,

Amber Mayes, Audrey Faust, and Cathy Vartuli. Your support during this process has meant the world to me.

And so much gratitude to Sara Connell and my Oracle friends. You know I couldn't have done this without your support.

To my Diamond Breakthrough Group: Nancy, Paula, Elsa, Miriam, Michèle and Linde. Here's to many more breakthroughs for all of us.

To my Before and After contributors: Sara Connell, Advait Shah, Christina Nylese, Debbie Forcier-Lynn, and Amanda Hinman. Thank you for your heart, courage, wisdom, and for your exceptional contributions to this book.

Thank you to my husband, John, who supported me through the highs and lows of this process (and there were many!). You know how grateful I am for your love and patience.

About the Author

Carol Look is a founding EFT master, licensed psychotherapist, best-selling author, international speaker, and creator of her signature coaching method, *The Yes Code*®. She combines her traditional training as a psychotherapist with clinical hypnosis and advanced applications of EFT for unprecedented results with her clients. Known for her laser-like focus and state of the art approach, Carol has used EFT for over 25 years to help clients release their limiting beliefs and emotional conflicts, so they can experience transformational changes and enjoy lives of exceptional success and fulfillment.

Carol is a world-renowned EFT workshop presenter and has taught workshops in England, the Netherlands, Belgium, France, Canada, Australia, and all over the United States. She is a regularly featured energy medicine expert on leading global summits, and is a featured expert in the field's documentaries: *The Tapping Solution*, *Leap*, and *Exploring Energy: The Ultimate Healer*. She has been invited to teach workshops for the Omega Institute, Kripalu, the Eden Energy Fest, and the energy field's primary teaching conference, ACEP.

Carol authored the original abundance book for the EFT field: *Attracting Abundance with EFT*, as well as *Improve Your Eyesight with EFT* and *Overcoming Overwhelm*. She is also known for creating downloadable Tapping Programs of the highest quality for practitioners and clients on the topics of success and abundance, weight loss, grief, PTSD, clearing clutter, and procrastination. Carol's most recent book, *The Yes Code*, became a number one best-seller on Amazon. For more on Carol's EFT programs, workshops, and books, please visit www.carollook.com and www.theyescode.com.

www.ingramcontent.com/pod-product-compliance
Lightning Source LLC
Chambersburg PA
CBHW070619030426
42337CB00020B/3849